community health nursing handbook

Mary Jo Clark, RN, MSN, PhD
Associate Dean
Associate Professor
Hahn School of Nursing and Health Science
University of San Diego
San Diego, California

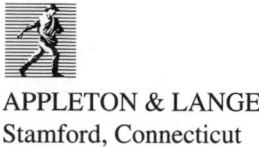

APPLETON & LANGE
Stamford, Connecticut

Notice: The author and the publisher of this volume have taken care to make certain that the doses of drugs and schedules of treatment are correct and compatible with the standards generally accepted at the time of publication. Nevertheless, as new information becomes available, changes in treatment and in the use of drugs become necessary. The reader is advised to carfully consult the instruction and information material included in the package insert of each drug or therapeutic agent before administration. This advice is especially important when using, administering, or recommending new or infrequently used drugs. The author and publisher disclaim all responsibility for any liability, loss, injury, or damage incurred as a consequence, directly or indirectly, of the use and application of any of the contents of this volume.

Copyright © 1999 by Appleton & Lange
A Simon & Schuster Company

All rights reserved. This book, or any parts thereof, may ot be used or reproduced in any manner without written permission. For information, address Appleton & Lange, Four Stamford Plaza, PO Box 120041, Stamford, Connecticut 06912-0041.

www.appletonlange.com

99 00 01 02 / 10 9 8 7 6 5 4 3 2

Prentice Hall International (UK) Limited, *London*
Prentice Hall of Australia Pty. Limited, *Sydney*
Prentice Hall Canada, Inc., *Toronto*
Prentice Hall Hispanoamericana, S.A., *Mexico*
Prentice Hall of India Private Limited, *New Delhi*
Prentice Hall of Japan, Inc., *Tokyo*
Simon & Schuster Asia Pte. Ltd., *Singapore*
Editora Prentice Hall do Brasil Ltda., *Rio de Janeiro*
Prentice Hall, *Upper Saddle River, New Jersey*

Clark, Mary Jo Dummer.
  Community health nursing handbook / by Mary Jo Clark.
    p. cm.
  ISBN 0-8385-1070-1 (pbk. : alk. paper)
  1. Community health nursing—Handbooks, manuals, etc.   I. Title.
  [DNLM: 1. Community Health Nursing handbooks.   WY 49C594c 1999]
  RT98.C5449 1999
  610.73'43—dc21
  DNLM/DLC
    for Library of Congress   98-37952
                                                              CIP

Acquisitions Editor: Patricia Casey
Associate Editor: Elisabeth Church Garofalo   ISBN 0-8385-1070-1
Production Editor: Angela Dion
Designer: Janice Barsevich Bielawa

PRINTED IN THE UNITED STATES OF AMERICA

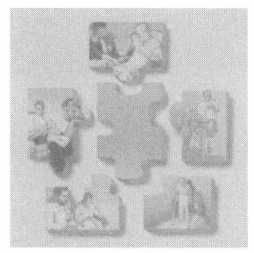

CONTENTS

Preface ....*ix*

Section I. The Dimensions Model of Community Health Nursing..... 1

The Dimensions Model of Community Health Nursing 1
Components of the Dimensions Model 2

Section II. The Process Dimension of Community Health Nursing 3

Health Promotion.. 3
  Nutritional Assessment Guide* / 4
  Effects of Selected Drug Classifications on Nutritional Status / 10
Health Education 11
  Tasks Involved in Planning a Health Education Encounter / 11
  Educational Planning and Implementation Guide* / 12
Home Visit 18
  Personal Safety Considerations in Home Visiting / 18
  Universal Precautions for Preventing the Spread of
    Bloodborne Diseases / 19
  Elements of a Home Visit / 20

* Indicates an assessment tool or inventory

iii

iv   CONTENTS

Home Safety Inventory / 21
Home Safety Inventory—Child* / 22
Home Safety Inventory—Older Person* / 24
Home Health Nursing Assessment* / 25

Case Management 31
Steps in the Case Management Process / 31
Components of the Referral Process / 32
Client Discharge Inventory* / 33
Resource File Entry Form* / 37

Group Process 40
Components of the Group Process / 40
Tasks of Group Development by Stage and Related Nursing Process Component / 41

Section III.   Influences on the Dimensions of Health 43

Cultural Influences 43
Modes of Cultural Exploration / 44
Cultural Assessment Guide* / 45

Environmental Influences 52
Common Poisonous Plants / 52
Primary Preventive Measures for Selected Environmental Hazards for Individuals, Families, and Communities / 53
Neighborhood/Community Safety Inventory* / 57

Section IV.   Care of Clients 61

The Child Client 61
Developmental Characteristics of Children of Selected Ages / 62
Anticipatory Guidance for Child Development / 64
Routine Screening of Children / 67
Recommendations for Routine Immunization—Children and Adults / 67
Newborn and Infant Reflexes / 68
Principles of Effective Discipline and Related Assessment Questions / 70

CONTENTS v

General Considerations in Assessing Children / 72
Questions for Assessing the Nutritional Status of Children
  of Selected Ages / 73
Child Health Assessment Guide* / 75
Primary Preventive Interventions in the Care of Children / 84
Nursing Interventions for Common Health Problems in Children / 85

The Adult Client 89
Developmental Characteristics of Adolescents and Adults / 89
General Considerations in Assessing Men's Health / 90
General Considerations in Assessing Women's Health / 91
Health Assessment Guide—Adult Client* / 92
Prenatal Care Checklist* / 101
Postpartum/Newborn Visit Intervention Checklist* / 105
Techniques for Teaching Breast Self-Examination (BSE) / 107
Techniques for Teaching Testicular Self-Examination (TSE) / 109

The Older Client 110
Common Physical Changes of Aging and Their Implications
  for Health / 110
Changes in Normal Laboratory Values in Older Clients / 114
General Considerations in Assessing Older Adults / 115
Functional Health Status Inventory* / 116
Cognitive Function Assessment Guide* / 120
Health Assessment Guide for the Older Client* / 123
Primary Prevention Strategies for Older Adults / 131
Secondary Prevention for Common Problems in Older Adults / 132
Principles of Reality Orientation / 134

The Family Client 135
Stages of Family Development / 135
Health Assessment and Intervention Planning Guide—
  Family Client* / 137
Family Crisis Assessment Guide* / 145

Population Groups 148
Sources of Community Assessment Data / 148
Health Assessment and Intervention Planning Guide—
  Community Client* / 150

Section V. Practice Settings 159

School Settings 159

Acute and Chronic Physical Health Problems Encountered in the School Setting / 160

Conditions Typically Warranting Exclusion from School and Guidelines for Readmission / 160

Health Assessment in the School Setting* / 162

Primary Prevention in the School Setting and Related Community Health Nursing Responsibilities / 170

Secondary Prevention in the School Setting and Related Community Health Nursing Responsibilities / 171

Tertiary Prevention in the School Setting and Related Community Health Nursing Responsibilities / 172

Work Settings 173

Health Hazards in Selected Occupational Settings / 173

Work Fitness Inventory*/ 176

Occupational Health Assessment Considerations / 180

Health Assessment in the Work Setting* / 181

Disaster Settings 189

Stages of Community Disaster Response / 190

Areas for Client Education Related to Disaster Preparedness / 191

Community Disaster Preparedness Checklist* / 192

Disaster Assessment and Planning Guide* / 193

Section VI. Common Community Health Problems 203

Communicable Diseases 203

Portals of Entry and Exit for Each Mode of Disease Transmission / 204

Information on Selected Communicable Diseases / 204

Communicable Disease Risk Factor Inventory* / 213

Communicable Disease Risk Factor Modification Strategies / 217

Chronic Physical Health Problems 218

Chronic Disease Risk Factor Inventory* / 219

Chronic Disease Risk Factor Modification Strategies / 222

Substance Abuse 224
    Fetal, Neonatal, and Developmental Effects of Perinatal Psychoactive
        Substance Exposure / 225
    Signs of Intoxication with Selected Psychoactive Substances / 226
    Indications of Withdrawal from Selected Psychoactive Substances / 227
    Substance Abuse Risk Factor Inventory* / 228
    Substance Abuse Risk Factor Modification Strategies / 231
    Treatment Modalities Typically Used for Selected Forms
        of Psychoactive Substance Abuse / 232
Violence 234
    Physical and Psychological Indications of Child Abuse / 234
    Physical and Psychological Indications of Spouse Abuse / 236
    Physical and Psychological Indications of Elder Abuse / 236
    Advantages and Disadvantages of Financial Arrangements to Prevent
        Financial Abuse of the Elderly / 238
    Family Violence Risk Factor Inventory* / 239
    Family Violence Risk Factor Modification Strategies / 242
    Suicide Risk Factor Inventory* / 244
    Suicide Risk Factor Modification Strategies / 247

Index *249*

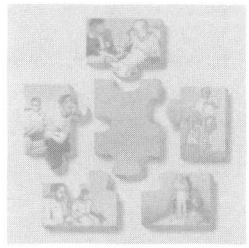

PREFACE

INTRODUCTION

In order to be useful in nursing practice, theoretical knowledge must be operationalized in specific activities to be performed by nurses to promote or restore the health of clients served. This is true of community health nursing knowledge as well as other areas of specialization. This handbook was written to assist community health nursing students and practicing community health nurses to translate the principles of practice into the actual care of individual, family, and community clients. It is intended to provide the reader with practical suggestions designed to enhance practice.

This handbook was written as a companion text to Clark's *Nursing in the Community: Dimensions of Community Health Nursing*, to provide a quick reference to information often needed by nurses in the field. It also contains several assessment guides and inventories that will assist the community health nurse or student to identify clients' health needs and design interventions to meet those needs. Many of the tools incorporated here are based on the Dimensions Model of community health nursing which is used as the organizing framework for *Nursing in the Community*. For practicing community health nurses, who already have a sound theoretical background, this book may be used alone. The community health nurse, however, may wish to refer to *Nursing in the Community* for an in-depth discussion of the Dimensions Model and its application to practice in the areas addressed by this handbook.

x PREFACE

ORGANIZATION

Community Health Nursing Handbook is organized in six sections, each related to a general area of community health nursing. Within each section, basic principles and information are presented for quick reference followed by assessment guides and inventories relevant to the section topic. Information is also provided on appropriate community health nursing interventions. A brief description of each section follows.

Section I: The Dimensions Model of Community Health Nursing

This section presents an overview of the Dimensions Model of community health nursing and describes the components of the model.

Section II: The Process Dimension of Community Health Nursing

This section presents information and assessment tools related to processes frequently used by community health nurses in their practice. Processes addressed include health promotion, health education, home visiting, case management, and the group process. Assessment guides and inventories are provided to assist the community health nurse to apply each process to the care of clients.

Section III: Influences on the Dimensions of Health

Although there are many factors in each of the six dimensions of health in the Dimensions Model that influence the health of individuals, families, groups, and communities, two are singled out here for in-depth discussion. The effects of cultural and environmental influences on health are presented along with assessment guides and inventories for guiding practice and suggestions for primary prevention by community health nurses.

Section IV: Care of Clients

Community health nurses provide care to a wide array of clients of all ages. Care is also provided to three levels of clients: individuals, families, and groups or communities. In this section, general assessment considerations are presented for several different types of clients including children, adult men and women, older clients, families, and population groups. Quick reference information and several assessment tools and inventories are also provided along with guidance for nursing interventions to deal with commonly encountered problems.

Section V: Practice Settings

Community health nurses practice in a variety of settings that present specific challenges and opportunities. Three of those settings—schools, work settings, and disaster settings—are presented here in terms of commonly encountered problems and relevant interventions. Assessment tools and inventories tailored to the needs of the setting are also provided. The section also provides guidance in planning for disaster response at the community level.

Section VI: Common Community Health Problems

Communicable diseases and chronic health problems, substance abuse, and violence are all significant public health problems in today's society. In this section, information related to these categories is presented in a quick reference format. Risk factor inventories and modification strategies for identified risk factors are also provided for communicable and chronic diseases, substance abuse, family violence, and suicide.

As noted earlier, most of the assessment guides and inventories are organized to reflect the six dimensions of health included in the Dimensions Model of community health nursing: the biophysical, psychological, physical, social, behavioral, and health systems dimensions. Each tool is preceded by a brief description of the tool; suggested populations, data sources, and data collection strategies; and purposes for which the information derived from the tool might be used. Many of the tools can be used with both individual and aggregate clients and provide direction for individual intervention or community-based health program planning. Copies of the actual tools are provided. These tools may be reproduced and used by the reader to collect information and guide practice in specific client situations.

In summary, the *Community Health Nursing Handbook* is intended as a quick-reference, practical guide to assist experienced community health nurses and those just learning the role to provide high quality, client-centered nursing care. It embodies the principles that have guided community health nursing practice for more than a century and that will continue to guide the profession in the next millennium.

Mary Jo Clark

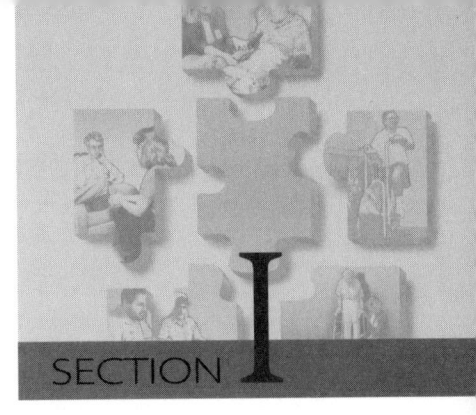

SECTION I

THE DIMENSIONS MODEL OF COMMUNITY HEALTH NURSING

▶ THE DIMENSIONS MODEL OF COMMUNITY HEALTH NURSING

The Dimensions Model of community health nursing combines public health science and nursing to create a model that can be used to direct community health nursing practice. The model incorporates an epidemiologic perspective and the concept of levels of prevention, interwoven with elements of nursing practice, to provide a framework for the use of the nursing process with individuals, families, and groups of people as the recipients of community health nursing services. See *Nursing in the Community: Dimensions of Community Health Nursing* (Chapter 5) for a complete discussion of the model.

▶ COMPONENTS OF THE DIMENSIONS MODEL

The Dimensions of Nursing: encompasses the knowledge, attitudes, values, and skills needed for community health nursing.

- Cognitive dimension: the knowledge base for community health nursing practice
- Interpersonal dimension: attitudes and values and interpersonal skills
- Ethical dimensions: ethical issues in practice
- Skills dimension: analytic skills (eg, critical thinking, diagnostic reasoning, data analysis) and manipulative skills (eg, catheterization, range of motion exercises)
- Process dimension: processes used by community health nurses
  Nursing process   Referral process
  Epidemiologic process   Change process
  Health education process   Leadership process
  Home visit process   Group process
  Case management process   Political process
- Reflective dimension: reflections on nursing care, includes evaluation, research, and theory development

The Dimensions of Health: factors affecting health status of individuals, families, and population groups

- Biophysical dimension: genetic inheritance, maturation and aging, and physiologic function
- Psychological dimension: psychological environmental influences on health (eg, coping, stress)
- Physical dimension: physical environmental influences on health (eg, safety hazards, weather)
- Social dimension: social environmental influences on health (eg, employment, poverty)
- Behavioral dimension: health-related behaviors (eg, alcohol use, seat belt use, BSE or TSE)
- Health system dimension: health system factors that influence health (eg, source of care, insurance)

The Dimensions of Health Care: levels of prevention at which community health nursing interventions occur

- Primary prevention: prevention of a health problem before it occurs
- Secondary prevention: resolution of an existing problem
- Tertiary prevention: prevention of complications of health problems or their recurrence, rehabilitation

SECTION II

THE PROCESS DIMENSION OF COMMUNITY HEALTH NURSING

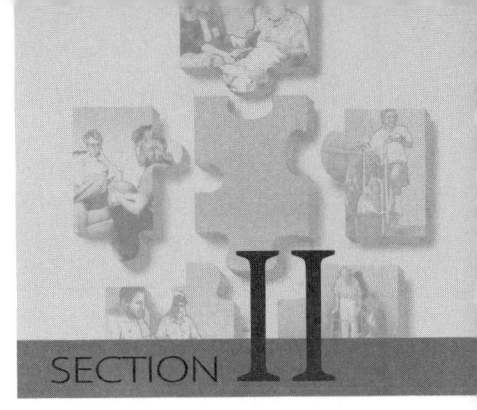

▶ HEALTH PROMOTION

A primary focus of community health nursing, health promotion, involves a wide range of activities designed to improve or maintain health. Health promotion entails responsibilities for both clients and nurses. Clients need to pursue health and health care actively by means of health-related behaviors. Nurses facilitate healthy behaviors by preparing clients to make behavioral choices that maximize their health potential. See *Nursing in the Community: Dimensions of Community Health Nursing* (Chapter 8) for a discussion of factors that promote health.

Because dietary practices profoundly influence well-being, adequate nutrition is a key aspect of health promotion. A well-balanced diet throughout life promotes normal growth and development and optimal health. The nurse assists the client (individual, family, or community) to identify and continue healthy dietary practices and to make dietary changes that promote health.

► NUTRITIONAL ASSESSMENT GUIDE

Description: Nutritional assessment involves interpretation of data from a variety of sources including anthropometric measurements, dietary history, physical examination findings, and the results of certain laboratory tests. Medication history and history of other behaviors (eg, alcohol intake) are also relevant to nutritional assessment because of potential nutritional effects (see the table of drug effects on nutritional status on page 10 of this handbook). Items contained in this tool are intended to assist the community health nurse to conduct a routine assessment of clients' nutritional status. They are framed in terms of the dimensions of health in the Dimensions Model. Items are *not* intended to support an in-depth nutritional assessment. In most cases, should an in-depth assessment be warranted, the community health nurse would refer the client to a nutritionist.

Appropriate populations: Individual clients of all ages.

Data sources and data collection strategies: Information can be derived from interviews with the client or significant others, from medical records, anthropometric measurements, medication review, and physical examination. The community health nurse may also observe clients' eating behaviors.

Use of information: Information obtained is primarily used as a basis for health education to promote nutritional health. Information may also give rise to nursing interventions or referrals for identified nutritional deficits or other problems (eg, obesity). Referrals may also be warranted for physical or psychosocial problems that interfere with optimal nutritional status (eg, difficulty swallowing or depression).

▶ NUTRITIONAL ASSESSMENT GUIDE

Biophysical Dimension Indicators of Nutritional Status

Height _____ Weight _____ Head circumference (< age 2 only) _____
Chest circumference (< age 2 only) _____

INDICATOR	YES	NO	DESCRIPTION
Unplanned weight loss > 10 lbs in 6 mos	☐	☐	
Recent weight gain	☐	☐	
Change in taste of foods	☐	☐	
Loss of appetite	☐	☐	
Increased appetite	☐	☐	
Food allergies	☐	☐	
Food intolerance	☐	☐	
Difficulty chewing	☐	☐	
Difficulty swallowing	☐	☐	
Poorly fitted dentures	☐	☐	
Sore mouth	☐	☐	
Toothache	☐	☐	
Choking	☐	☐	
Dietary restrictions	☐	☐	
Problems with food preparation ability	☐	☐	
Fatigue	☐	☐	
Fever lasting longer than 3 days	☐	☐	
Diarrhea	☐	☐	
Constipation	☐	☐	
Nausea	☐	☐	
Vomiting	☐	☐	
Dry mouth	☐	☐	
Belching	☐	☐	
Heartburn	☐	☐	
Flatulence	☐	☐	
Indigestion	☐	☐	
Increased urination	☐	☐	
Decreased urination	☐	☐	
Increased thirst	☐	☐	
Pregnancy	☐	☐	
Decubiti	☐	☐	
Recent surgery	☐	☐	

INDICATOR	YES	NO	DESCRIPTION
Crohn's disease or ulcerative colitis	☐	☐	
Chronic liver disease	☐	☐	
Chronic renal failure	☐	☐	
Cancer	☐	☐	
Diabetes	☐	☐	
Hypertension	☐	☐	
Cardiovascular disease	☐	☐	
Thyroid disease	☐	☐	
Anemia	☐	☐	
Hypercholesterolemia	☐	☐	
Mobility limitations	☐	☐	

Physical Dimension Indicators of Nutritional Status

	YES	NO
Inadequate facilities for food preparation	☐	☐
Inadequate facilities for food storage	☐	☐

Psychological and Social Dimension Indicators of Nutritional Status

	YES	NO
Depression	☐	☐
Mental retardation or mental illness	☐	☐
Confusion or disorientation	☐	☐
Alzheimer's disease	☐	☐
Social isolation	☐	☐
Inadequate food budget	☐	☐
Religious food prescriptions or proscriptions	☐	☐

Cultural food preferences: _____

_____

Behavioral Dimension Indicators of Nutritional Status

Fluid intake (*amount, type, frequency*): _____

Favorite foods: _____
Foods disliked: _____
Use of laxatives, cathartics, etc.: _____

Smoking habits: _____
Alcohol or other drug use (*amount, type, frequency, duration*): _____

Food preparation practices: _____
Meal patterns (*frequency, timing, amount eaten*): _____

General food intake:

CATEGORY	DAILY SERVINGS	SERVING SIZE	USUAL TYPE
Grains and cereals			
Fruits			
Vegetables			
Milk and milk products			
Red meats and pork			
Poultry, fish, legumes, nuts			
Eggs			
Iron-rich foods			
Other foods (butter, sugar, etc.)			

8 COMMUNITY HEALTH NURSING HANDBOOK

Daily diet history

DAY OF WEEK:		
Morning meal Food	Time eaten: Amount eaten	Typical: Yes ____ No ____
Midday meal Food	Time eaten: Amount eaten	Typical: Yes ____ No ____
Evening meal Food	Time eaten: Amount eaten	Typical: Yes ____ No ____
Snack Food	Time eaten: Amount eaten	Typical: Yes ____ No ____
Snack Food	Time eaten: Amount eaten	Typical: Yes ____ No ____
Snack Food	Time eaten: Amount eaten	Typical: Yes ____ No ____

MEDICATION USE*	YES	NO
Antacids	☐	☐
Antibiotics	☐	☐
Anticoagulants	☐	☐
Anticonvulsants	☐	☐
Antidepressants	☐	☐
Antihypertensives	☐	☐
Antineoplastics	☐	☐
Antituberculins	☐	☐
Aspirin	☐	☐
Cathartics	☐	☐
Diuretics	☐	☐
Hypocholesterolemics	☐	☐
Oral contraceptive agents	☐	☐
Sedatives/hypnotics	☐	☐
Steroids	☐	☐

Health System Indicators of Nutritional Status

Therapeutic diet prescribed: _____
Radiation therapy: _____
Chemotherapy: _____

Nutrition-related Health Problems Identified:

1. _____
2. _____
3. _____
4. _____
5. _____

Nursing Interventions for Nutrition-related Problems:

1. _____
2. _____
3. _____
4. _____
5. _____

---

* Not all drugs in these categories have nutritional effects, and nutritional effects may vary among drugs in the same category. The community health nurse should familiarize him- or herself with the particular effects of specific drugs in each category.

▶ EFFECTS OF SELECTED DRUG CLASSIFICATIONS ON NUTRITIONAL STATUS

DRUG CLASSIFICATION	EFFECTS
Alcohol	May cause GI upset. May also affect thiamine, vitamin B_{12}, folate, magnesium, and zinc levels.
Aspirin	May cause GI upset. May also affect protein metabolism, vitamin K and C, and potassium levels.
Antacids	May affect thiamine, phosphorus, and iron levels.
Antibiotics	May cause GI upset and anorexia. May also affect protein, carbohydrate, and fat metabolism, vitamin A, D, K, riboflavin, vitamin B_{12}, B_6, folate, vitamin C, calcium, iron, sodium, potassium, magnesium, and zinc levels.
Anticoagulants	May affect vitamin K levels.
Anticonvulsants	May cause anorexia. May also affect vitamin D, B_{12}, B_6, folate, calcium, and magnesium levels.
Antidepressants	May cause GI upset. May also affect carbohydrate metabolism, calcium, and magnesium levels.
Antihypertensives	May cause GI upset and anorexia. May also affect vitamin B_6, calcium, sodium, and potassium levels.
Antineoplastics	May cause GI upset and anorexia. May also affect protein, carbohydrate, and fat metabolism, vitamin B_{12}, and folate levels.
Antituberculins	May affect protein, carbohydrate, and fat metabolism, niacin, vitamin B_{12}, B_6, folate, calcium, iron, and magnesium levels.
Cathartics	May affect carbohydrate metabolism, vitamin A, D, K, calcium, phosphorus, and potassium levels.
Diuretics	May affect carbohydrate metabolism, thiamine, B_6, folate, calcium, potassium, magnesium, and zinc levels.
Hypercholesterolemics	May cause GI upset. May also affect carbohydrate and fat metabolism, vitamin A, D, K, B_{12}, folate, calcium, iron, sodium, and potassium levels.
Oral contraceptives	May cause GI upset. May also affect protein metabolism, riboflavin, vitamin B_{12}, B_6, folate, vitamin C, magnesium, and zinc levels.
Sedatives/hypnotics	May affect riboflavin, phosphorus, sodium, potassiums and magnesium levels.
Steroids	May cause GI upset and weight gain. May also affect protein, carbohydrate, and fat metabolism, vitamin D, B_6, folate, vitamin C, calcium, phosphorus, potassium, and zinc levels.

▶ HEALTH EDUCATION

Much of the practice of community health nursing involves educating people about healthier lifestyles. Health education enables people to make decisions regarding personal behaviors, their use of health resources, and their position on societal issues that affect health.

The health education process consists of assessing the learner and the learning situation, diagnosing learning needs, and planning, implementing, and evaluating a health education presentation. In planning a health education encounter, the community health nurse will establish priorities for health education, identify goals, develop learning objectives, select content and teaching strategies, prepare educational materials, and develop a plan to evaluate the lesson. See *Nursing in the Community: Dimensions of Community Health Nursing* (Chapter 9) for an in-depth discussion of the health education process.

▶ TASKS INVOLVED IN PLANNING A HEALTH EDUCATION ENCOUNTER

Identifying the Goal
- Specifying the broad purpose to be accomplished

Developing Objectives
- Stating specific behavioral outcomes expected as a result of the encounter

Classifying Objectives
- Identifying the learning domains to be addressed

Selecting and Sequencing Content
- Determining what will be taught and the order in which it will be presented

Selecting Teaching Strategies
- Determining approaches to be used in presenting content

Preparing Materials
- Developing any teaching aids to be used in the presentation

Planning Evaluation
- Determining criteria and processes to be used for formative, outcome, and process evaluation

▶ EDUCATIONAL PLANNING AND IMPLEMENTATION GUIDE

Description: In order to educate clients to make appropriate health-related decisions, community health nurses must identify health learning needs and then design health education encounters that address those needs and that take into account the three major elements of the learning situation, client characteristics, the material to be learned, and the setting in which learning is to take place. The tool presented here is designed to assist the community health nurse to assess clients' health education needs and to plan effective health education encounters to meet those needs.

Appropriate populations: Individual clients of all ages, groups of clients with similar learning needs.

Data sources and data collection strategies: The assessment data collected using the *Educational Planning and Implementation Guide* can be obtained from a number of sources. Much information about clients can be obtained in interviews with clients or significant others or from a review of existing health, school, or other records. Information regarding health learning needs may be derived from knowledge of existing physical conditions that create a need for specific learning or from learning needs typical of clients' ages. Learning needs may also be identified in interviews or client surveys or through pretesting in specific content areas. Assessment of client maturation may be derived via interviews, by observation, or from developmental testing. Information about motivation to learn and other psychological factors affecting the learning situation can be obtained from interviews, records, and by observing clients' responses to the learning situation. Behavioral data is best obtained in interviews with clients or significant others or by actual observation of client behaviors. Information about the physical environment in which the learning encounter is to take place is most often available through direct observation. Attitudes to health and health care or to specific health education topics may be assessed through interviews, client surveys, or the use of attitude scales. Social dimension information such as education level, income, culture, religion, occupation, and so on, may be available in existing records or can be obtained directly from clients through interviews and surveys, and information about health system factors can be derived in similar ways.

Use of information: Educational assessment data allow the community health nurse to identify clients' learning needs and factors that influence the learning situation. This information then leads to delineation of specific outcome objectives for the health education encounter. Teaching strategies are selected that are appropriate to the content, to client characteristics, and to other factors that influence the learning situation. After employing these strategies in a planned educational encounter, the community health nurse evaluates learning in terms of the established outcome objectives for the encounter. Outcome evaluation may involve testing for knowledge gained, attitude assessment, or observation of learner behaviors, depending on the intended learning outcomes. The nurse also evaluates the quality of the educational assessment and the materials and strategies used.

▶ EDUCATIONAL PLANNING AND IMPLEMENTATION GUIDE

Client: _____ Phone: _____
Address: _____
Contact person (for group encounters): _____

Assessment of Learning Situation

Biophysical Dimension
Client age(s): _____ Sex: _____ Race: _____
Possible influence of physical maturation on learning: _____

Physical conditions giving rise to health education needs: _____

Physical conditions that might influence ability to learn: _____

Psychological Dimension
Readiness and motivation to learn: _____

Psychological factors that may impede learning (*stress, anxiety, depression, confusion, disorientation*): _____

Coping abilities: _____

Physical Dimension
Physical environmental conditions giving rise to health education needs: __

Physical environment for learning (*noise, light levels, distractions*): _____

Social Dimension
Education level: _____
Socioeconomic level: _____
Religion: _____
Ethnicity: _____
Primary language: _____
Facility with English: _____
Cultural influences on the learning situation: _____
Social support for healthy behavior (*peer interactions, role models*): _____

Occupation(s): _____

Behavioral Dimension

Nutrition (food consumption, preferences, preparation): _____

Other consumption patterns: _____

Health-related behaviors:
    Immunizations: _____
    Exercise: _____
    Dental hygiene: _____
    Seat belt use: _____
    Other safety precautions: _____
    Contraceptive use: _____
    Sexual activity: _____

Health Care System

Access to health care: _____
Knowledge of health care resources: _____
Use of health-promotive services: _____
Use of restorative/rehabilitative services: _____
Attitudes to health and health care: _____

▲ PLANNING AND IMPLEMENTING THE HEALTH EDUCATION ENCOUNTER

EDUCATIONAL DIAGNOSES	LEARNING OBJECTIVES	CLASSIFICATION OF LEARNING OBJECTIVES	TEACHING STRATEGIES	EVALUATION PLAN

▶ EVALUATION OF HEALTH EDUCATION ENCOUNTER

Evaluation of Learning Outcomes

OBJECTIVE	STATUS MET/UNMET	EVIDENCE

Process evaluation: _____

_____
_____
_____
_____

Revisions needed: _____

_____
_____
_____
_____
_____

▶ HOME VISIT

Historically a major focus of community health nursing, today the home is only one of many settings where community health nurses provide care for clients. Despite the broadening of community health nursing to encompass a multitude of settings, the home visit process remains a strategic tool for health care delivery. A home visit, as conceptualized in community health nursing, is a formal call by a nurse on a client at the client's residence to provide nursing care.

The advantages to making home visits are many. Home visits permit health care services to be integrated into the client's usual routine. For clients who are immobile or lack transportation, the home visit affords access to health care that might otherwise be unavailable. The nurse making a home visit may gather information about the client and the client's environment less easily obtained in other settings, including information about resources and hazards, the extent of the client's support network, and the client's ability to perform activities of daily living. In many cases, home visits are more economical and result in better outcomes than care provided in other settings.

Home visiting presents challenges as well as advantages. Challenges arise from a diverse population with multiple health problems and from the need to maintain balance between opposing pressures, including needs for intimacy and distance, dependence and independence, and cost-containment and quality of care. See *Nursing in the Community: Dimensions of Community Health Nursing* (Chapter 10) for an in-depth discussion of the home visit process.

▶ PERSONAL SAFETY CONSIDERATIONS IN HOME VISITING

Appearance

- Wear a name tag and a uniform or other apparel that identifies you as a nurse
- Do not carry a purse or wear expensive jewelry
- Leave any valuables at home or lock them in the trunk of the car

Transportation

- Keep your car in good repair and with a full tank of gas
- Carry emergency supplies such as a flashlight and blanket
- Always lock your car and carry keys in hand when leaving the client's home

- Park near client's home with your car in view of home whenever possible
- Avoid the use of public transportation, if possible
- Get complete and accurate directions to the home

The Situation

- Call ahead to alert the client that you will be coming
- Ask clients to secure pets before your visit
- Walk directly to the client's home, without detours to local shops or other places
- Keep one arm free while walking to the client's home
- Avoid isolated areas, especially late in the day
- Knock before entering the client's home, even if the door is open
- Make joint visits in dangerous neighborhoods or situations or employ an escort service if needed
- Listen to the client's messages regarding potential safety hazards
- Make home visits at times when illicit activity (such as drug transactions) is less likely to occur or when potentially dangerous family members will not be present
- Carry a whistle that is easily accessible
- Become familiar with personal defense techniques
- Leave any situation that appears to hold a risk of personal danger
- Stay alert and observe your surroundings

▶ UNIVERSAL PRECAUTIONS FOR PREVENTING THE SPREAD OF BLOODBORNE DISEASES

- Use appropriate barrier precautions (eg, gloves) to prevent skin and mucous membrane exposure when contact with human blood or other body fluids is anticipated
- Wash hands and other skin surfaces immediately after contamination with blood or other body fluids
- Take precautions to prevent injuries stemming from needles and other sharp instruments during or after procedures, when disposing of used equipment, or when cleaning used equipment
- Do not recap, bend, or break used needles; place them in a puncture-proof container for disposal
- Keep mouthpieces, resuscitation bags, or other ventilation devices at hand when the need for resuscitation is predictable
- Refrain from direct care of clients and from handling client care equipment when you have exudative skin lesions or weeping dermatitis

20 COMMUNITY HEALTH NURSING HANDBOOK

- Implement these precautions with all clients, not just those known to be infected with bloodborne diseases

Source: Recommendations for prevention of HIV transmission in health care settings. (1988). MMWR, 36(Suppl 2), 35–185.

▶ ELEMENTS OF A HOME VISIT

Preparatory assessment	Review available client data to determine health care needs related to biophysical, psychological, physical, social, behavioral, and health system dimensions
Diagnosis	Develop diagnostic hypotheses based on preparatory assessment
Planning	Review previous interventions and their effects
	Prioritize client needs and identify those to be addressed during the visit
	Develop goals and objectives for visit and identify levels of prevention involved
	Consider client acceptance and timing of visit
	Specify activities needed to accomplish goals and objectives
	Obtain needed supplies and equipment
	Plan for evaluation of the home visit
Implementation	Validate preparatory assessment and nursing diagnostic hypotheses
	Identify other client needs
	Modify plan of care as needed
	Carry out nursing interventions
	Deal with distractions
Evaluation	Evaluate client response to interventions
	Evaluate long-term and short-term outcomes of intervention
	Evaluate the quality of implementation in the home visit
Documentation	Document client assessment and health needs identified
	Document interventions
	Document client response to interventions
	Document outcome of interventions
	Document future plan of care

SECTION II THE PROCESS DIMENSION OF COMMUNITY HEALTH NURSING 21

▶ HOME SAFETY INVENTORY

Description: The two tools presented here are designed to assist the community health nurse to identify safety hazards in the home.

Appropriate populations: The tools are designed specifically for use with children and older adults, respectively, but can be modified for use with other clients. For example, the *Home Safety Inventory—Older Adult* could be used to assess the safety of the home situation for a client with a disability. Similarly, the *Home Safety Inventory—Child* could be used to assess environmental safety in a child-care setting. Many of the items are also relevant to home safety for all clients whatever their age or health status and can be used to identify general safety hazards present in the home or other settings.

Data sources and data collection strategies: Information on areas addressed by the *Home Safety Inventory* tools can be obtained by interviews with clients, parents, or other family members or by observation of the home setting.

Use of information: The results of either inventory can be used to educate individual clients or families regarding home safety issues and to motivate changes in environmental conditions to promote safety in the home. The inventories can also be completed by groups of people and the results used to initiate home safety education.

▶ HOME SAFETY INVENTORY—CHILD

AGE	SAFETY CONSIDERATION	YES	NO
Infant	1. Safe sleeping arrangements made for infant?	☐	☐
	2. Parents aware of bathing safety (not leaving child unattended, water temperature)?	☐	☐
	3. No loose parts on toys?	☐	☐
	4. Approved car restraint used consistently?	☐	☐
	5. Infant seat left on elevated surfaces?	☐	☐
	6. Infant restraint straps consistently used in infant seat, stroller, high chair, car seat?	☐	☐
	7. Small objects kept out of reach?	☐	☐
Toddler/ preschool child	1. Poisons, sharp objects, etc., kept locked away?	☐	☐
	2. Poisonous substances stored in appropriate containers?	☐	☐
	3. Childproof lids correctly placed on medications and other toxins?	☐	☐
	4. Medications stored in locked area?	☐	☐
	5. Gates/barriers placed on stairs?	☐	☐
	6. Safety locks present on doors and upstairs windows?	☐	☐
	7. Child closely supervised at play?	☐	☐
	8. Child supervised at all times during bath?	☐	☐
	9. Toys have no small parts?	☐	☐
	10. Electrical outlets covered?	☐	☐
	11. Electrical cords left dangling?	☐	☐
	12. Pots and pans placed toward back of stove with handles turned toward rear?	☐	☐
	13. Play equipment in good repair?	☐	☐
	14. Outdoor play area is fenced and gates locked?	☐	☐
	15. Outdoor play area has resilient surface?	☐	☐
	16. Poisonous plants present in home or yard?	☐	☐
	17. Car seat belt used consistently?	☐	☐

AGE	SAFETY CONSIDERATION	YES	NO
	18. Caution used and taught in crossing streets?	☐	☐
School-age child	1. Child supervised in sports and outdoor play?	☐	☐
	2. Play equipment free of safety hazards?	☐	☐
	3. Outdoor play area floored with sand, shavings, or wood chips?	☐	☐
	4. Firearms kept locked with key inaccessible?	☐	☐
	5. Bicycle helmet worn consistently?	☐	☐
	6. Children taught not to open door to strangers?	☐	☐
	7. Car seat belt used consistently?	☐	☐
Adolescent	1. Firearms safety taught?	☐	☐
	2. Firearms stored unloaded with safety lock on?	☐	☐
	3. Teen cautioned not to admit being home alone?	☐	☐
	4. Car seat belt used consistently?	☐	☐

▶ HOME SAFETY INVENTORY—OLDER PERSON

SAFETY CONSIDERATION	YES	NO
1. Lighting adequate on stairs?	☐	☐
2. Stair rails present and in good repair?	☐	☐
3. Nonskid surfaces on stairs?	☐	☐
4. Throw rugs present safety hazard?	☐	☐
5. Crowded living area presents safety hazard?	☐	☐
6. Tub rails installed?	☐	☐
7. Tub has nonslip surface?	☐	☐
8. Space heaters present safety hazard?	☐	☐
9. Adequate provision made for refrigeration of food?	☐	☐
10. Medications kept in appropriately labeled containers with readable print?	☐	☐
11. Toxic substances have labels with readable print and are stored well away from food?	☐	☐
12. Home is adequately ventilated and heated?	☐	☐
13. Neighborhood is safe?	☐	☐
14. Fire and police notified of older person in home?	☐	☐

▶ HOME HEALTH NURSING ASSESSMENT

Description: This tool is designed to assess the health needs of clients who are receiving community health nursing services in the home setting.

Appropriate populations: Any client receiving home nursing services including those provided by a home health nursing agency.

Data sources and data collection strategies: Assessment information included in the tool may be obtained by interviewing the client or significant others, by review of existing health records, in conversation or in writing from referring health care providers, or through physical examination and direct observation.

Use of information: Assessment data is used to design nursing interventions appropriate to the home as a setting for care.

► HOME HEALTH NURSING ASSESSMENT

Patient name: _____ Birth date: _____ Record #: _____
Address: _____
Phone number: _____

Biophysical Dimension

Male _____ Female _____
Primary medical diagnosis: _____
Past medical history: _____
_____

General appearance: _____
_____

Vital signs: Temp: _____ Pulse: Apical _____ Radial: _____ Respirations: _____
Weight: _____ Height: _____
Blood pressure: 1) Right arm—Supine _____ Sitting _____ Standing _____
              2) Left arm—Supine _____ Sitting _____ Standing _____
Hearing: Normal _____ Hearing impaired: _____ Deaf: _____
        Uses hearing aid: R _____ L _____
Vision: Normal _____ Blind: _____ Limited: _____
Uses glasses: Sometimes _____ Always _____

Developmental level: _____
Allergies: _____

Functional abilities: No problems: _____ Difficulty with: Bathing _____
Dressing _____ Toileting _____ Mobility/transfer _____ Eating _____
Bowel control _____ Bladder control _____ Communication _____
Meal preparation _____ Housekeeping _____ Shopping _____
Use of assistive devices: _____
Describe any limitations noted: _____
_____

Immunization status: _____

Review of Systems

Neurological: No problems _____ Oriented x _____ Headache _____
Vertigo _____ Tremors _____ Seizures _____ Syncope _____
Parasthesias _____ Weakness _____
Level of Consciousness (LOC) (describe): _____
_____

Cardiovascular: No problems _____ Palpitations _____ Fainting _____
Dizziness _____ Edema _____ Cyanosis _____
Neck vein distention _____ Chest pain _____ Pulse irregularity _____
Syncope _____ Circumoral pallor _____

Respiratory: No problems _____ Dyspnea _____ SOB _____ SOBOE _____
Orthopnea _____ Cough _____ Cyanosis _____ Pain _____ Sputum _____
IPPB _____ O_2 _____
Lung sounds (describe) _____

Gastrointestinal: No problems _____ Nausea _____ Vomiting _____
Anorexia _____ Bleeding _____ Pain _____ Diarrhea _____
Constipation _____ Incontinent _____ Distention _____ Aphagia _____
NGT _____ GT _____ JT _____ Bowel sounds (describe) _____

Genitourinary: No problems _____ Frequency _____ Urgency _____
Pain _____ Burning _____ Nocturia _____ Hematuria _____
Difficulty urinating _____ Incontinent _____ Retention _____
Catheter _____

Integumentary: No problems _____ Cool _____ Warm _____
Diaphoresis _____ Pallor _____ Cyanosis _____ Flushing _____
Mottling _____ Jaundice _____ Pruritis _____ Petechiae _____ Dry _____
Decubitus _____ Pressure areas _____
Wound/incision (describe) _____
Rash (describe) _____
Bruises (describe) _____
Turgor (describe) _____

Musculoskeletal: No problems _____ Joint swelling _____
Decreased ROM _____ Back pain _____

Reproductive: No problems _____ Impotence _____ Prostatitis _____
Discharge _____ Breast mass _____ Testicular mass _____
Decreased libido _____ Dysmenorrhea _____ Dyspareunia _____
Last Pap smear: _____

Hematopoietic: No problems _____ Anemia _____ Epistaxis _____
Bruising _____ Venous access: Good _____ Fair _____ Poor _____

Immunologic: Frequent infection _____ Diminished immune status _____
HIV infection _____

Pain: None _____ Description _____

Intensity: 1+ (mild) _____ 2+ (discomfort) _____ 3+ (distressing) _____
4+ (severe) _____ 5+ (excruciating) _____
Analgesics taken _____ Dose _____ Frequency _____
Effectiveness _____
Degree of limitation due to pain _____

Psychological Dimension

Mood: No problems _____ Depressed _____ Anxious _____ Restless _____
Uncooperative _____
Mentation: Alert _____ Confused _____ Disoriented _____
Coping: Adequate _____ Minimal _____ Inadequate _____
History of mental illness: _____
Recent loss: _____
Life satisfaction: _____
History of family violence: _____
Sources of stress: _____
_____

Physical Dimension

Type of residence: House _____ Apartment _____ Institution _____
  Shelter _____ None _____
Ease of access: Stairs to climb _____ Ramp _____
Space: Adequate _____ Inadequate: _____
Distance to bathroom: _____
Home safety: Adequate _____
Safety hazards present: _____
Safety features in home: Childproof latches _____ Tub rail _____
  Grounded outlets _____ Stair lights _____ Stair rails _____
  Smoke alarm _____
Infection control hazards: _____
Inadequate: Lighting _____ Heat _____ Ventilation _____
  Air conditioning _____ Refrigeration _____ Cooking facilities _____
  Plumbing _____ Waste disposal _____ Electricity _____
Use of space heaters: _____
Storage of hazardous materials: _____
Firearms in home: _____
Home maintenance/repair: Adequate _____ Inadequate _____
Describe problems noted: _____
Pets: Type _____ Indoor _____ Outdoor _____
Neighborhood safety: _____
Environmental pollutants: _____

Social Dimension

Education level: _____ Income: _____
Primary language: _____ Interpreter: _____
Religious affiliation: _____ Ethnicity: _____
Employed _____ Unemployed _____ Retired _____
Occupation(s): _____
Single _____ Married _____ Divorced _____ Widowed _____
Other persons in home: (include ages, health problems, etc.) _____

Quality of family interactions: _____

Opportunity for social interaction: _____

Social support network: _____

Cultural influences: _____

Availability of transportation: _____

Behavioral Dimension

Diet: Inadequate in: Calories _____ Protein _____ Iron _____
  Potassium _____ Calcium _____ Vitamin A _____
  Vitamin B complex _____ C _____ D _____ K _____ Fluid _____
  Fiber _____ Excessive Fat _____ Calories _____ Sodium _____
Method of preparation: _____
Typical meal pattern: _____

Other substances: Alcohol use _____ Amount _____
Illicit drug use _____ Type _____ Amount _____ Route _____
Tobacco use _____ Type _____ Amount _____
Length of use _____
Medications (include prescription and over-the-counter medications):
   Medication   Dose   Frequency   Route   Purpose   Length of use
1.
2.
3.
4.
5.
Sleep patterns: _____

Exercise: _____

Leisure activities: _____

Sexually active: _____ Orientation: _____
Satisfaction: _____
Unsafe sexual practices: _____

Other behaviors: Seat belt use _____ Contraceptive use _____ BSE/TSE _____
Use of other safety equipment: _____

Health System Dimension

Usual source of health care: _____
Source of health care funding: _____
Use of preventive services: _____
Attitudes to health and health care: _____
Barriers to access: _____

▶ CASE MANAGEMENT

As practiced by community health nurses, case management is a process of identifying needs for and arranging, coordinating, monitoring, and evaluating quality, cost-effective health care services to achieve designated outcomes. Case management affords advantages for both the client and the health care industry, including better coordination of care, minimizing confusion about a complex health care system, providing access to acceptable and affordable health care services, attention to multiple health care needs, improving health outcomes, minimizing hospitalization, preventing rehospitalization, and eliminating duplication of services.

Effective case management programs are client- and family-centered, utilize a multidisciplinary, multiservice approach along a continuum of care, and are collaborative, cooperative, outcome-oriented, and resource efficient. See *Nursing in the Community: Dimensions of Community Health Nursing* (Chapter 11) for an in-depth discussion of the case management process.

▶ STEPS IN THE CASE MANAGEMENT PROCESS

Assessing the Dimensions of Health
- Biophysical dimension
- Psychological dimension
- Physical dimension
- Social dimension
- Behavioral dimension
- Health system dimension

Deriving Nursing Diagnoses

Developing the Case Management Plan
- Determining levels of prevention
- Selecting resources

Implementing the Case Management Plan
- Communicating the plan
- Initiating referrals
- Monitoring plan implementation

Evaluating the Process and Outcomes of Case Management
- Evaluating primary, secondary, and tertiary intervention outcomes
- Evaluating the quality of services

- Evaluating the case management process
- Utilization review

▶ COMPONENTS OF THE REFERRAL PROCESS

Assessment
- Assess referral needs in terms of:
    Biophysical factors
    Psychological factors
    Physical factors
    Social factors
    Behavioral factors
    Health system factors
- Assess acceptability of referral to client
- Assess client eligibility for service
- Identify situational constraints

Diagnosis
- Diagnose the need for referral
- Diagnose client care needs to be met by referral resources

Planning
- Establish goals and objectives of referrals for primary, secondary, or tertiary preventive services
- Select appropriate referral resources
- Prepare client for the referral
- Plan follow-up

Implementation
- Provide client with information needed to follow through with referrals
- Communicate with agencies and providers regarding client needs

Evaluation
- Evaluate outcomes of referral for primary, secondary, and tertiary preventive services
- Evaluate the referral process

▶ CLIENT DISCHARGE INVENTORY

Description: Case management is often initiated when clients are being discharged from a health care facility or institution with continuing care needs. The tool presented here is intended to be used to identify client discharge needs and to direct planning to meet those needs.

Appropriate populations: Clients being discharged from an acute care setting to community health nursing services, or clients being discharged from community health nursing services to other agencies or to self-care.

Data sources and data collection strategies: Data needed for effective discharge planning are available from several sources including interviews with clients, significant others, or health care personnel; health records; or observation of the client.

Use of information: Assessment data are used to identify areas in which assistance is required and to identify the care to be provided as well as appropriate sources of that care.

► CLIENT DISCHARGE INVENTORY

Biophysical Dimension

Name: _____ Age: _____
Sex: _____ Race/ethnicity: _____
Indicate the extent to which the client needs assistance and the type of assistance needed with each of the following functions:

AREA OF FUNCTION	TYPE OF ASSISTANCE NEEDED	TO BE PROVIDED BY
Bathing		
Dressing		
Eating		
Elimination		
Mobility		

Does the client have medical diagnoses that require follow-up?

MEDICAL DIAGNOSIS	TYPE OF FOLLOW-UP NEEDED	TO BE PROVIDED BY

Is the client on any medications? Do these medications give rise to needs for care?

MEDICATION	CARE NEEDED	TO BE PROVIDED BY

Does the client have physical impairments that affect self-care abilities? ___

Does the client have other biophysical needs that necessitate care? ___

Psychological Dimension

Does the client's emotional/mental status give rise to needs for care? ___

What stresses does the client experience? ___

Is the client able to cope effectively? ___

Physical Dimension

Discharge address: ___
Are there physical hazards in the discharge environment? If so, describe them: ___

Social Dimension

Describe the client's social support network: ___

Are there cultural influences affecting client needs for care? ___

Does the client have needs related to the following socioeconomic concerns?

AREA OF NEED	TYPE OF ASSISTANCE NEEDED	TO BE PROVIDED BY
Finances		
Transportation		
Social interaction		
Shopping		
Child care		
Occupation		

Behavioral Dimension

Do any of the following health-related behaviors give rise to needs for care?

BEHAVIOR	TYPE OF ASSISTANCE NEEDED	TO BE PROVIDED BY
Alcohol use		
Diet		
Drug use		
Leisure activity		
Safety measures		
Smoking		

Health System Dimension

What level(s) of services are needed from the health care system?

LEVEL OF PREVENTION	TYPE OF SERVICE NEEDED	TO BE PROVIDED BY
Primary		
Secondary		
Tertiary		

▶ RESOURCE FILE ENTRY FORM

Description: This tool is designed to assist the community health nurse to obtain pertinent data about available community resources. Many of the notations are self-explanatory, but several warrant explanation. The "resource category" notation, for example, refers to the type of agency or category of service provided (eg, transportation, financial assistance, etc.). Funding sources may be public funds or tax dollars, private donations, fee-for-service, and so on. The contact person is a person in the agency to whom the community health nurse is known and who may be able to assist the nurse's clients with a minimum of "red tape." The "source of referral" entry reflects persons or agencies from whom referrals for services are accepted. For example, some agencies require that clients be referred by a primary health care provider, others accept self-referrals. The "eligibility" entry addresses criteria that clients must meet to be eligible for services. These may include residence in a particular area, certain age groups, or financial indigency. An entry should also be made regarding any fees that clients may be required to pay as well as what sources of payment are accepted (eg, insurance, Medicaid). The "services" entry describes specific services provided by the agency, while "access" reflects the means by which clients gain access to the service agency. For example, whether or not an appointment is needed and how it is obtained. "Other comments" would include any other relevant information about the agency that would influence community health nursing referrals.

Appropriate populations: Community agencies. May include health-related agencies and those that are only indirectly involved in influencing the health of clients (eg, employment services). Information obtained could be targeted to agencies providing certain categories of services (eg, services to children) or to a broad range of community services that may be of use to community health nurses and their clients.

Data sources and data collection strategies: Basic information about an agency may be derived from telephone book listings (eg, name, address, telephone number) or from existing area service directories, where available. Service directories are often out-of-date, so information should be confirmed in a telephone or personal contact with key agency personnel. These contacts can also elicit information that may not be included in standard service directories. Entries under "other comments" may include comments from prior clients regarding the services provided or past experiences of community health nurses in dealing with the agency. This information is best obtained in interviews with those persons who have had interactions with the service agency. Information obtained should be updated on a regular basis (at least annually, or as information changes). The community health nurse may find it helpful to maintain a key contact person in each agency who will alert the nurse to changes in agency services or policies.

Use of information: Community health nurses use the information contained in the *Resource File Entry Form* to plan and implement referrals that are appropriate to a given client's situation and needs. Use of this information allows the nurse to eliminate inappropriate referrals that are frustrating for clients and service personnel.

▶ RESOURCE FILE ENTRY FORM

Resource category: _____ Funding source: _____
Agency name: _____
Address: _____
Phone number: _____ Business hours: _____
Contact person: _____ Title: _____
Source of referral: _____
Eligibility: _____
_____
Fee: _____
Services: _____
_____
_____
_____
_____
_____
_____
Access: _____
Other comments: _____
_____
_____
_____
_____

▶ GROUP PROCESS

Change, particularly within the health care delivery system, is often accompanied by group action. Community health nurses are often called upon to initiate and direct group problem-solving activities, as well as to serve in groups formed by others. In contrast to individual efforts, group action affords a broader base of knowledge and expertise and promotes communication that may enhance problem resolution.

Group development occurs in a series of stages, and specific tasks must be accomplished during each stage for the group to function effectively. See *Nursing in the Community: Dimensions of Community Health Nursing* (Chapter 12) for an in-depth discussion of group process.

▶ COMPONENTS OF THE GROUP PROCESS

Assessment	Assess the problem to be addressed by the group
	Assess the members of the group in terms of factors influencing group function:
	• Biophysical dimension
	• Psychological dimension
	• Physical dimension
	• Social dimension
	• Behavioral dimension
	• Health system dimension
Diagnosis	Diagnose group strengths and weaknesses, expertise, and motivation
Planning	Plan achievement of group goals
	Plan group operation in terms of:
	• Methods for group decision making
	• Mechanisms for conflict resolution
	• Methods of communication
	• Role negotiation
Implementation	Implement activities designed to reach the group goal
	Implement group operation procedures
Evaluation	Evaluate outcome of the group action
	Evaluate use of the group process

▶ TASKS OF GROUP DEVELOPMENT BY STAGE AND RELATED NURSING PROCESS COMPONENT

NURSING PROCESS COMPONENT	STAGE OF GROUP DEVELOPMENT	GROUP DEVELOPMENT TASKS
Assessment	Orientation	1. Selection of group members 2. Training for group participation 3. Identification of goals and purposes
Diagnosis		
Planning	Accommodation	1. Establishment of modes of decision making 2. Development of mechanisms for conflict resolution 3. Development of communication network 4. Development of climate conducive to group collaboration
	Negotiation	1. Negotiation of member roles 2. Development of methods of task assignment
Implementation	Operation	1. Assignment of specific tasks to accomplish group goals 2. Performance of actions to accomplish goals
Evaluation	Dissolution	1. Planning of evaluative mechanisms for outcomes of action taken 2. Assignment of member roles and tasks in evaluation 3. Data collection 4. Analysis of evaluative findings 5. Possible group dissolution

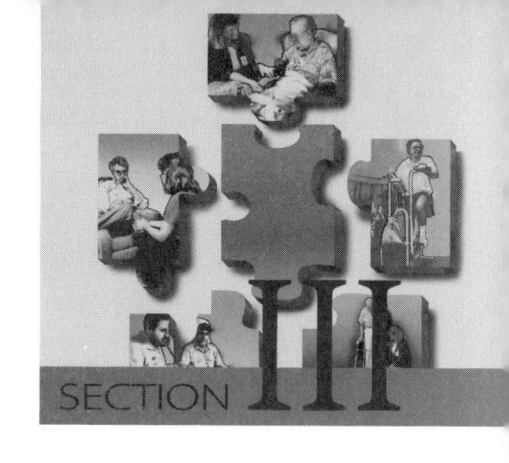

INFLUENCES ON THE DIMENSIONS OF HEALTH

▶ CULTURAL INFLUENCES

Community health nurses, like the clients they serve, come from a wide variety of cultural backgrounds. Without knowledge of culture and its influences on daily life and health, cultural differences experienced by community health nurses and their clients can lead to ineffective nursing care. Culturally relevant care, on the other hand, can enhance the effectiveness of community health nursing. It is, therefore, particularly important for community health nurses to consider their clients' cultural backgrounds in formulating care to meet their needs.

Respect and acceptance of differences in cultural beliefs, values, and behaviors facilitate the rapport required by the level of intimacy between nurse and client that characterizes community health nursing. The nurse's knowledge of cultural factors can facilitate communication, allow more accurate identification of potential health problems, and enhance the potential for compliance via an intervention plan tailored to the client's lifestyle.

At the aggregate level, culturally relevant care has implications beyond health. By planning and implementing culturally relevant health care programs, the community health nurse conveys respect for and acceptance of multiple cultural groups and sets the stage for greater cohesion and cooperation in society-at-large. See *Nursing in the Community: Dimensions of Community Health Nursing* (Chapter 16) for an in-depth discussion of cultural influences on health.

▶ MODES OF CULTURAL EXPLORATION

- Become conversant with your own culture and its influences on your life.
- Review the existing literature on beliefs, values, and behaviors of specific cultural groups.
- Interview colleagues who are members of the cultural group in question.
- Immerse oneself in the culture to be studied.
- Observe members of specific cultural groups.
- Interview members of cultural groups, particularly group leaders.
- Interview other persons who are conversant with the culture.

▶ CULTURAL ASSESSMENT GUIDE

Description: This tool is intended to assist the community health nurse to assess another culture and to give him or her a better understanding of the effects of culture on health. The tool is framed in terms of the six dimensions of health included in the Dimensions Model of community health nursing, and data are collected relative to the biophysical, psychological, physical, social, behavioral, and health system dimensions. Development of positive, health-promotive, and problem-focused nursing diagnoses that can guide intervention with the cultural group is emphasized. The guide concludes with entries related to specific nursing interventions that are appropriate to the cultural group assessed and activities that should be avoided.

Appropriate populations: Any cultural group, even the nurse's own culture.

Data sources and data collection modes: Information about another culture is available from a number of sources. You might want to begin your search with the literature describing the culture of interest. The literature of several disciplines should be examined including health-related literature, psychological and sociological literature, anthropological literature, and educational literature. Information about the culture may also be gleaned from its literary works and its art. Other sources of data are interviews with members of the cultural group and should include people of different ages to gain a perspective on changes that may be occurring in the culture with time. Observation and participation in cultural events and in everyday life within the culture are other ways of gleaning information about another culture. Health professionals who are members of the culture of interest may also be able to provide you with insights even if they do not themselves engage in behaviors typical of the cultural group. Clients who are members of another cultural group are also sources of information about their beliefs, values, and behaviors.

Use of information: Information gleaned in assessing another culture provides an understanding of the behavior of others and provides the nurse with guidance in planning culturally sensitive and relevant nursing intervention. Designing nursing interventions around clients' own beliefs, values, and behaviors increases the potential for effective health care and client compliance with health recommendations.

▶ CULTURAL ASSESSMENT GUIDE

Cultural group to be assessed: _____

Biophysical Dimension

What is the age composition of the cultural group? _____
How is age viewed in the culture? _____
At what age are group members considered adults? _____
Are there cultural rituals associated with coming of age? _____

Do group members display distinctive physical features? _____

Do group members display differences in normal physiologic parameters (eg, height, weight, hematocrit)? _____

What genetically determined illnesses are present in the group? ____

What are the cultural attitudes to body parts and physiologic functions? Are some body parts to be kept covered? _____

What bodily functions are considered private? _____

Are there specific culturebound syndromes recognized by the group? ____

What scientific medical diagnoses are prevalent in the group? _____

Psychological Dimension

What are the cultural attitudes to mental health and illness? _____

What behaviors are considered aberrant by group members? _____

Are individual or group goals more important? _____

How is authority exercised? By whom? What are group members' attitudes to authority? _____

What is the group's attitude to change? _____
What is the quality of interaction between the cultural group and the dominant society? _____

Physical Dimension

Has the group been physically isolated from the dominant society? _____

What are group members' attitudes toward nature? _____

Do environmental hazards pose particular risk for group members (eg, pesticide exposure in migrant farm workers)? _____

Social Dimension

Interpersonal Relationships

What is the typical family structure? _____
What roles are typical of family members? _____

How interchangeable are roles? _____
How congruent are culturally-prescribed roles with those of the dominant society? _____

Communication

What is the primary language spoken? _____
How important is context to communication? _____
Are there formal and informal modes of address? How are they used? _____

Is personal reticence characteristic of group members? _____

What courtesy titles are used? for whom? _____

What gestures are considered appropriate? inappropriate? _____

Demeanor

What behaviors are expected in interactions with others? _____

What behaviors are unacceptable? _____

Beliefs and Values

What are the group's basic value orientations to:

- Human nature? _____

- Natural environment? _____
- Time? _____
- Activity? _____
- Relationships? _____

What value do group members place on:

- Health? _____
- Material gain? _____
- Punctuality? _____
- Education? _____
- Individualism? _____

What values are given priority in the culture? _____

Religion and Magic
What is(are) the typical religious affiliation(s)? _____
Does religion influence health? How? _____

Are religious leaders involved in health care? How? _____

What is the effect of religious sponsorship on use of health services? ____

Are religious beliefs and practices incorporated into health care? How? ___

Do group members express belief in magical causes of disease or cure? ___

Economic Status
What is the economic status of group members? _____

What occupations are typical of group members? _____

Behavioral Dimension

Dietary Patterns
What are the typical food preferences and consumption patterns? _____

How are foods usually prepared? _____
Do certain foods have special symbolism? _____

SECTION III INFLUENCES ON THE DIMENSIONS OF HEALTH   49

Are certain foods used to prevent or cure illness? What are they? _____
_____
Are there nutrients typically lacking in group members' diets? _____
_____

Other Consumption Patterns
What are group attitudes to use of:

- Alcohol? _____
- Tobacco? _____
- Other drugs? _____
- Caffeine? _____

To what extent are these substances used or abused by group members? __
_____

Life events
What are group attitudes to conception? _____
To contraception? _____
Is conception expected early in marriage?_____
Are there cultural practices to promote or prevent conception? _____
_____
Are certain behaviors expected in pregnancy?_____
_____
Are certain behaviors avoided during pregnancy? _____
_____
What is the attitude to prenatal care?_____
Are there cultural practices related to labor and delivery?_____
_____
Who should be present during labor and delivery? _____
_____
Where should labor and delivery occur? _____
Are there special practices related to disposal of the placenta? ___
_____
What behaviors are expected in the postpartum period? _____
_____
What are the care practices for the newborn? Who executes them? ___
_____
What are group attitudes to breastfeeding? _____
What are group attitudes to death? _____
Do group members want to know of terminal conditions? _____
_____
Is there belief in an afterlife? _____
Where should death occur? _____

Who should be present at the time of death? _____

Who should prepare the body? _____
How is the body disposed of? _____
Are there practices related to grief and mourning? _____

Who should participate in rituals and practices related to death? _____

Sexual Practices

What are group attitudes to homosexuality? _____

What are group attitudes to heterosexual activity? _____

Do group members engage in specific sexual practices? _____

Do members practice female genital mutilation? _____

Health System Dimension

How are health and illness defined? _____

What theories of disease causation are held? _____

Are there recognized folk health practitioners? Who are they? How do they learn their craft? _____
_____

What health promotive, preventive, diagnostic, and treatment measures do folk practitioners employ? _____
_____
_____

To what extent are folk health practitioners used? _____

What primary preventive measures are used by group members? _____

What secondary preventive measures are used? _____

Are any folk health practices used potentially harmful? _____

What is the relationship of folk and scientific health care systems within the group? _____

To what extent do group members use both systems? _____

Positive Nursing Diagnoses Related to the Group

1. _____
2. _____
3. _____
4. _____
5. _____

Health-promotive Nursing Diagnoses Related to the Group

1. _____
2. _____
3. _____
4. _____
5. _____

Problem-focused Nursing Diagnoses Related to the Group

1. _____
2. _____
3. _____
4. _____
5. _____

Culturally Relevant Nursing Interventions

1. _____
2. _____
3. _____
4. _____
5. _____

Activities to Be Avoided, if Possible

1. _____
2. _____
3. _____
4. _____
5. _____

▶ ENVIRONMENTAL INFLUENCES

Environmental factors influence human health and welfare. Air, water, noise, radiation, and waste present a variety of hazards to human health. Environmental conditions present three types of hazards: physical, biological, and chemical or gaseous. Community health nurses are concerned with the effects of environmental hazards on the health of individuals, families, and communities, and interventions may occur at any of these levels. See *Nursing in the Community: Dimensions of Community Health Nursing* (Chapter 17) for an in-depth discussion of environmental factors as they influence health.

▶ COMMON POISONOUS PLANTS

Arrowhead vine
Asparagus fern
Azalea
Begonia
Chrysanthemum
Climbing nightshade
Dumbcane
"Fiesta" pepper
Firethorn
Flame violet
Holly
Honeysuckle
Jade plant
Jerusalem cherry
Medicine aloe
Mistletoe
Mountain-ash
Oak
Oleander
Oregon grape
Philodendron
Poinsettia
Poison ivy
Pokeweed
Rhododendron
Rubber plant
Schefflera
Spiderplant
Weeping fig tree

▶ PRIMARY PREVENTIVE MEASURES FOR SELECTED ENVIRONMENTAL HAZARDS FOR INDIVIDUALS, FAMILIES, AND COMMUNITIES

ENVIRONMENTAL HAZARD	INDIVIDUAL/ FAMILY	COMMUNITY
Radiation	Refer for assistance with testing and sealing a home against radon leaks	Educate the public on the hazards of radon exposure and preventive measures
	Encourage spending most of one's time in higher levels of the home	Engage in political activity to promote standards that safeguard occupants in areas with high levels of natural radiation
	Discourage overuse of diagnostic x-rays	Educate public about the hazards of overuse of diagnostic x-rays
	Encourage adequate cleaning of door seals on microwave ovens and maintenance of safe distance while microwave is in operation	Engage in political activity to promote and enforce safety standards for nuclear reactors
	Discourage sunbathing Encourage use of sunscreen and protective clothing when outdoors	Educate public about hazards of exposure to ultraviolet radiation
Lead and heavy metals	Encourage families to have lead-based paint removed from older homes	
	Encourage families to wash hands of young children as well as toys to remove lead-contaminated dust	
	Encourage close supervision of young children	

ENVIRONMENTAL HAZARD	INDIVIDUAL/ FAMILY	COMMUNITY
	Encourage families to use cold water to drink and cook with and to allow the tap to run for a few minutes	Promote legislation to ban air pollution and acid rain to prevent pollution of water with heavy metals Encourage policy makers to set and enforce standards for solid waste sites to prevent metal contamination in water
Noise	Encourage families to limit noise in the home Encourage use of ear protection in high-noise areas	Promote noise abatement ordinances
Infectious agents	Promote routine immunization for all ages	Educate the public on need for immunization Encourage policy makers to provide low-cost immunization
	Encourage good hygiene	
	Encourage washing fruits and vegetables before eating	
	Encourage adequate refrigeration of food	Encourage enforcement of regulations for food processing and food handlers
	Encourage susceptible individuals to boil water for cooking and drinking in areas with unsafe water	Promote adequate sanitation, waste disposal, and water treatment
Insects and animals	Encourage immunization of family pets	Encourage development and enforcement of immunization and leash laws

SECTION III INFLUENCES ON THE DIMENSIONS OF HEALTH

ENVIRONMENTAL HAZARD	INDIVIDUAL/ FAMILY	COMMUNITY
	Refer for help in eliminating insects, rats, and other pests from the home Encourage use of insect repellent and protective clothing when outdoors	Promote ordinances controlling insect breeding areas
Plants	Eliminate poisonous house plants Eliminate poisonous plants from the yard Eliminate other hazardous plants (eg, poison ivy, plant allergens) from home environment Encourage close supervision of children	Eliminate poisonous plants from recreational areas
Poisons	Educate families on proper use and storage of household chemicals and medications Encourage close supervision of children	Educate public on hazards of household chemicals and medications Promote legislation to limit use of hazardous chemicals in home and industry
Air pollution	Encourage limiting physical activity on days with high air pollutant levels Encourage car-pooling Discourage use of space heaters in poorly ventilated areas Encourage frequent cleaning of heater and air-conditioning filters	Promote legislation to prevent air pollution Promote legislation to develop safety standards for home heating devices Promote building standards that ensure adequate ventilation

ENVIRONMENTAL HAZARD	INDIVIDUAL/ FAMILY	COMMUNITY
	Encourage opening doors and windows to permit air exchange Encourage replacing asbestos insulation as needed	
Water pollution	Encourage use of bottled water by high risk persons in areas with heavily polluted water	Promote legislation to prevent water pollution

▶ NEIGHBORHOOD/COMMUNITY SAFETY INVENTORY

Description: This tool can be used to assess physical and psychosocial safety hazards in a client's neighborhood or in a community-at-large. The tool assesses elements of the physical, psychological, and social dimensions of health in the Dimensions Model. The inventory promotes identification of safety problems in the neighborhood or community and planning of nursing interventions to resolve identified problems.

Appropriate populations: Any neighborhood or community.

Data sources and data collection strategies: Personal observation of the neighborhood and interviews with residents and key informants are excellent means of obtaining information about neighborhood or community safety. Examples of key informants include local police and fire personnel, business and industry leaders, community officials, local disaster planning groups, department of transportation officials, and insurance company representatives. Review of police, fire, and insurance records may also be a source of important environmental safety information.

Use of information: Information derived using the tool can be used to educate individual clients regarding elimination or avoidance of safety hazards. Information may also be helpful in planning community safety education programs, in initiating disaster planning efforts, or to support political activity to enhance neighborhood or community safety. Finally, neighborhood safety information may assist the nurse to take precautions to promote his or her own safety while working in the area. Using information derived from the inventory, the community health nurse develops nursing diagnoses related to safety problems and plans interventions for those problems. Frequently, the interventions needed will require collaboration with other agencies and individuals, but may be initiated by the nurse.

▶ NEIGHBORHOOD/COMMUNITY SAFETY INVENTORY

Neighborhood or community assessed:_____

Safety Hazards in the Natural Environment

What is the extent of air pollution? What pollutants are involved? _____

What is the extent of water pollution? What pollutants are involved?_____

What is the extent of natural radiation in the area? _____

Are there other environmental pollutants in the area? _____

Do local weather conditions pose health hazards? _____
Are there drowning hazards (eg, lakes, rivers) in the area? _____
Do wild animals in the area serve as reservoirs for disease? _____
What poisonous plants or plant allergens grow in the area? _____

Safety Hazards in the Constructed Environment

Do residential units pose safety hazards? _____

What is the extent of disrepair in housing units?_____
Are there structural defects in area buildings, roads, etc., that pose safety hazards? _____

Do local building codes effectively address safety issues? _____
Are building safety codes enforced? _____
Is there a lead exposure hazard in the area? _____
How adequate is sanitation and waste disposal?_____
What is the prevalence of residential fires? _____
What proportion of homes in the area have functional smoke alarms or sprinkler systems?_____
What are the local fire insurance rates? _____
To what extent do residents (home owners and renters) carry fire insurance? _____

What is the response time for fire personnel? _____
Are area swimming pools adequately fenced?_____
What is the prevalence of traffic accidents? Do they tend to occur in specific areas? _____
What are the local car insurance rates? _____

To what extent do residents carry automobile insurance? _____
What is the response time for emergency personnel? _____
Are there significant noise hazards in the area? _____
What safety hazards are posed by local industry? _____

To what extent do local industries adhere to safety standards? _____

Safety Hazards in the Psychological Environment

How secure do area residents feel? _____
To what extent do environmental conditions contribute to stress? _____

Safety Hazards in the Social Environment

What is the extent of crime in the area? What types of crime are involved?

What is the response time for police personnel? _____
Do area residents take an active part in crime prevention? _____
What is the extent of intergroup conflict in the area? _____

Is there tension between racial or ethnic groups in the area? _____

Is there gang violence in the area? _____
What is the extent of family violence in the area? _____

What is the response of protective services personnel to episodes of family violence? _____

What is the extent of drug and alcohol use/abuse in the area? _____

Are drug dealers a problem in the area? _____
What is the extent of drug-related crime in the area? _____

Disaster Potential

What is the potential for flooding? _____
What is the potential for earthquake? _____
What is the potential for brush fires or forest fires? _____
What is the potential for toxic exposures? _____
What is the potential for explosions? _____
Is there a community disaster plan? Are area residents aware of the plan?

Neighborhood/Community Safety Problems Identified:

1. _____
2. _____
3. _____
4. _____
5. _____

Nursing Interventions to Address Safety Problems:

1. _____
2. _____
3. _____
4. _____
5. _____

SECTION IV

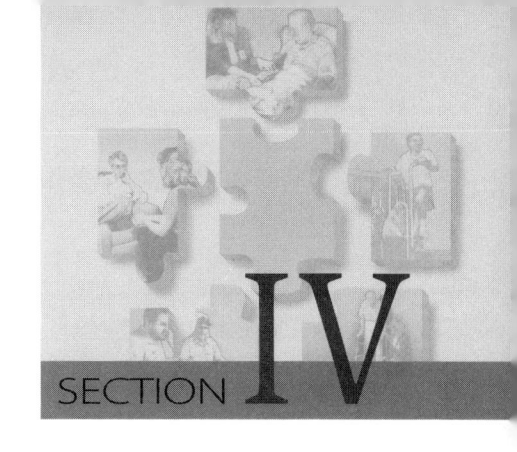

CARE OF CLIENTS

▶ THE CHILD CLIENT

Care of children presents community health nurses with significant opportunities to influence the future health of the general population. One of the most effective ways to improve the health status of a community is to maintain and enhance the health of its children. Health promotion and prevention for this age group can make a tremendous impact on the overall future health of a population. Children who receive effective health care services, particularly health promotion and illness prevention services, are far less likely to develop a variety of acute and chronic health problems. If children are taught to engage in healthy behaviors, their lifetime health status will be positively influenced. See *Nursing in the Community: Dimensions of Community Health Nursing* (Chapter 20) for an in-depth presentation of care for children.

▶ DEVELOPMENTAL CHARACTERISTICS OF CHILDREN OF SELECTED AGES

AGE		DEVELOPMENTAL CHARACTERISTIC
Birth–1 month	Neurophysical	Newborn reflexes intact, head lag present, follows objects to midline, responds to noise
	Psychosocial	Regards human face, quiets when picked up
1–2 months	Neurophysical	Follows objects 180°, holds head up in prone position, head erect and bobbing when supported in sitting position
	Psychosocial	Vocalizes other than crying, smiles responsively
2–4 months	Neurophysical	Newborn reflexes diminishing, sits well with support, rolls from side to side, grasps rattle
	Psychosocial	Laughs aloud, initiates smiling, enjoys play activity
4–6 months	Neurophysical	Reaches for and gets objects, puts objects in mouth, rolls over completely, supports own weight when standing, tooth eruption
	Psychosocial	Turns to voice, begins stranger anxiety, strong attachment to caretaker
6–9 months	Neurophysical	Sits alone, bounces, stands holding on, thumb–finger grasp
	Psychosocial	"Mama" or "dada," plays peek-a-boo and pattycake, imitates speech sounds
9–12 months	Neurophysical	Pulls to stand, creeps or crawls, walks holding on, sits from standing position, uses a cup with help
	Psychosocial	Gives toy on request, speaks two to three words, gives affection, indicates wants
12–18 months	Neurophysical	Scribbles, points to one or more body parts, uses a spoon, climbs and runs, plays ball, beginning bowel training
	Psychosocial	Likes to be read to, 10-word vocabulary

AGE		DEVELOPMENTAL CHARACTERISTIC
18–24 months	Neurophysical	Opens doors, turns on faucets, can throw or kick a ball, walks up and down stairs alone, daytime bowel and bladder control established
	Psychosocial	Parallel play, 2–3 word sentences, imitates household tasks
2–3 years	Neurophysical	Dresses with help, rides a tricycle, washes and dries hands
	Psychosocial	Separates easily from mother, uses pronouns, perceives danger, understands sharing and taking turns
3–5 years	Neurophysical	Dresses with decreasing supervision, hops on one foot, catches bounced ball, heel-to-toe walk
	Psychosocial	Gives whole name, recognizes three colors, draws person with more than six parts, tells a story, operates from rules
5–10 years	Neurophysical	Physical growth slows, motor coordination increases
	Psychosocial	Begins peer identification, forms friendships, learns more rules, begins sexual identification, increases use of language to convey ideas, begins to understand cause and effect
11–14 years	Neurophysical	Begins pubertal changes, gawkiness
	Psychosocial	Importance of peer group conformity, strong identification with members of the same gender, learning one's role in heterosexual relationships, begins to establish an identity, more abstract thought, negative attitude to family

▶ ANTICIPATORY GUIDANCE FOR CHILD DEVELOPMENT

DEVELOPMENTAL ISSUE	ANTICIPATORY GUIDANCE
Rolling over	Do not place child on elevated surface. Place child prone on blanket on floor while awake.
Sitting	Support head and shoulders until head control achieved.
Teething	Use a cold teething ring to promote comfort (or tie an ice cube in a washcloth). Do not use teething preparations or alcohol on gums. Begin cleaning teeth with a washcloth or soft toothbrush after first tooth errupts.
Feeding self	Allow child to feed self finger foods. Allow practice with spoon even if it makes a mess (place a plastic sheet under high chair and place high chair in shower to wash off excess food, if needed). Feed child at table with others who can be observed eating. Allow child to hold cup with help. Mash small foods (eg, peas, etc.) to prevent choking or placing in ears, nose, etc. Supervise child during meals.
Creeping and crawling	Allow child safe place to creep. Keep small objects off floor. Cover electrical outlets. Remove dangling cords.
Standing and walking	Pad sharp corners of furniture. Keep external doors closed and latched. Place gates at head of stairs. Avoid use of baby "walkers."
Hand–mouth movement	Remove small objects and detachable parts of toys to prevent choking. Wash hands and toys frequently, expecially in high lead areas.
Weaning	Use cup at mealtimes. May still take bottle before being put down for nap or at night, but do not put child in bed with bottle. Put only water, not milk, in nap or bedtime bottle.
Exploration	Keep all poisons and sharp objects locked up. Childproof cabinets. Store medications, cleaning supplies, etc., appropriately. Provide close supervision of young children.

DEVELOPMENTAL ISSUE	ANTICIPATORY GUIDANCE
	Hold child's hand when walking across streets and in parking lots.
	Teach street safety, stranger safety.
Climbing	Do not put unsafe objects up high. Provide close supervision of children.
Negativity	Present choices among options, not a choice of whether to do or not do something. For example, ask the child "Do you want to put on your pajamas or brush your teeth first?" rather than "Let's put on your pajamas." Ignore frequent "no" answers.
Decreased appetite	Normal with slowed rate of growth. Feed several small meals and snacks. Finger foods that can be eaten "on-the-go" (with adequate supervision) tolerated well. Give small portions and allow child to ask for more, if desired. Vary colors and textures. Give nutritious foods for meals and snacks; avoid junk foods.
Toilet training	Watch for signs of readiness (walking, increasing time between wet diapers, squatting, pulling at wet or dirty diaper).
	Identify elimination pattern and put child on potty seat for short periods at identified times.
	Take child to toilet immediately on request; they cannot wait.
	Praise appropriate elimination. Do not punish for mistakes.
	Nighttime accidents may occur until school age. Do not shame child if accidents occur. Limit fluids after dinner. Empty bladder just before bed. Wake child to urinate just before parents go to bed. If bedwetting persists beyond age 6, seek assistance.
Speech	Talk to child, encourage vocalization. Read to child.
	For children who are late talking, make sure others are not meeting needs before they are voiced. Discourage parents and siblings from responding to grunts, pointing, and crying. Encourage child to say what it is he or she wants.

DEVELOPMENTAL ISSUE	ANTICIPATORY GUIDANCE
Night terrors	Place a night light in room. Provide "protector" stuffed animal. If child awakens in night, comfort, show safety of room, and put back to bed in own room.
Separation anxiety	Explain need for parent to leave. Leave with well-known persons. Reassure of parental return. Allow child to speak to parent on phone during extended absence. Maintain familiar surroundings, favorite toys, etc.
Dressing self	Give child opportunities to dress self. Provide minimal help as needed.
Bedtime resistance	Develop and engage in regular bedtime ritual. Do not rock or hold child until he or she falls asleep. If child gets up, return him or her to bed. Can place safe toys in bed with child and allow play until he or she falls asleep.
Sibling rivalry	Treat all children fairly. If oldest child has extra privileges, explain why to younger children. If other conditions warrant differential treatment, explain why.
School anxiety	Assist child to make friends at school. Assist with homework. Praise sincere effort and small successes. Engage in learning games.
Sexual development	Discuss sexuality with preadolescent. Discuss wet dreams with boys, menstruation with girls, and conception with both boys and girls.
Values testing	Allow adolescents to make choices and then experience the consequences. Try to maintain open lines of communication with frank discussion of issues such as drug and alcohol use, sexuality, etc. Maintain limits on behavior, while permitting increasing independence.

SECTION IV CARE OF CLIENTS   67

▶ ROUTINE SCREENING OF CHILDREN

AGE	SCREENING TEST
Birth	Phenylketonuria (PKU), T_4
6 months	Hematocrit or hemoglobin, lead
9 months	Tuberculin skin test (PPD)
1 year	Hematocrit or hemoglobin, sickle cell (for African Americans), lead
2 years	Hematocrit or hemoglobin
3–4 years	Hematocrit or hemoglobin, lead, blood pressure, hearing, vision, dental
5–6 years	Hematocrit or hemoglobin, lead, blood pressure, hearing, vision, dental, urinalysis (for girls)
7–8 years	Hematocrit or hemoglobin, lead, blood pressure, hearing, vision, dental
9–10 years	Hematocrit or hemoglobin, lead, blood pressure, hearing, vision, scoliosis, dental
11–12 years	Hematocrit or hemoglobin, lead, blood pressure, hearing, vision, scoliosis, dental

▶ RECOMMENDATIONS FOR ROUTINE IMMUNIZATION—CHILDREN AND ADULTS

IMMUNIZING AGENT	RECOMMENDATIONS FOR ADMINISTRATION
Diphtheria, tetanus, pertussis vaccines (DTP)	2, 4, 6, and 18 months, school entry
Tetanus, diphtheria vaccine (Td)	Children over 7; adults: booster every 10 years
Trivalent inactivated poliovirus vaccine (IPV)	Healthy children: 2 and 4 months Immunocompromised children: 2, 4, and 18 months, and at school entry
Trivalent oral poliovirus vaccine (OPV)	Healthy children: 18 months, school entry
Measles, mumps, rubella vaccine (MMR)	15 months, booster at school entry
Haemophilus influenzae type B vaccine (HiB)	2, 4, and 6 months; booster at 15 months

IMMUNIZING AGENT	RECOMMENDATIONS FOR ADMINISTRATION
Hepatitis B vaccine (HBV)	Children: birth, 1 month, 6 months Health care workers, prostitutes, others with multiple sexual partners, injection drug users: an initial dose followed by a second dose 1 month later and a third dose 6 months later
Varicella vaccine	Children: one dose given between 12 months and 12 years of age Persons 13 years of age or older: two doses, 4–8 weeks apart
Influenza vaccine	Annually for persons over age 65 and those with debilitating physical illness
Pneumonia vaccine	Persons over age 65 and those with debilitating physical illness

▶ NEWBORN AND INFANT REFLEXES

REFLEX	DESCRIPTION	APPEARS	DISAPPEARS
Asymmetrical tonic neck	Assumption of a "fencing" position when head is turned to side. Face is toward extended arm and leg, other arm and leg flexed.	1–2 months	By 6 months
Laundau	Elevation of the head and arching of spine in prone position.	9–12 months	By 36 months
Moro (startle)	Pattern varies, but usually involves symmetrical abduction of upper extremities, extension of elbow and fingers, then movement of hands toward each other and return to flexion	Birth	By 6 months (weakens gradually)

REFLEX	DESCRIPTION	APPEARS	DISAPPEARS
	in response to loud noise or sudden lowering of the supine body rapidly about 12 inches.		
Neck righting	Rotation of shoulders, trunk, and pelvis in the same direction, moments after active or passive rotation of head (immediate response is abnormal).	4 months	Persists
Optical placing of hands	Forward extension of extremities and dorsiflexion of hands when infant is rapidly dropped in prone position and allowed to see drop. Sometimes confused with parachute reflex.	May be as early as 3 months	Persists
Palmar grasp	Curling of fingers around examiner's finger placed in palm of hand.	Birth	By 6 months (usually earlier)
Parachute	Forward extension of extremities and dorsiflexion of hands when rapidly dropped in prone position with attention distracted from seeing drop.	6–12 months	Persists
Plantar grasp	Curling of toes around examiner's finger placed at base of toes.	Birth	8–9 months (may persist in sleep for a short while longer)
Rooting and sucking	Turning face toward finger stroking cheek, sucking motion.	Birth	3–4 months (may persist in sleep until 7–8 months)

REFLEX	DESCRIPTION	APPEARS	DISAPPEARS
Supporting reaction	Increased weightbearing when held upright with feet touching firm surface.	About 4 months	Replaced by voluntary standing by 10–11 months.
Traction response	Ability to support head and neck when pulled slowly from supine to sitting position.	Well established by 6–7 months	Persists

▶ PRINCIPLES OF EFFECTIVE DISCIPLINE AND RELATED ASSESSMENT QUESTIONS

Principle 1: Determine What Is Important

- Have parents determined what behaviors are never acceptable?
- Is there a good rationale for this determination?
- Do parents say "no" automatically?

Principle 2: Be Consistent

- Are parents consistent in what is considered unacceptable behavior?
- Do parents allow children to wear them down until they let unacceptable behavior pass?
- Do parents agree on what behavior is unacceptable, or can children manipulate parents?
- Have parents determined situations in which certain behavior, otherwise acceptable, is not allowed?
- Have parents explained to children the reason for the difference in what is allowable at some times and not at others?

Principle 3: Never Act in Anger

- Do parents control their anger?
- Do parents use a "cooling off" period when needed?
- Have parents explained the reason for the cooling off period so children will learn appropriate ways of dealing with anger?

Principle 4: Allow Time for Compliance

- Do parents allow time for children to comply with directions, or do they expect instant obedience?

- Do parent's respect children's needs to complete a task in which they are engaged before complying with parental instructions?

Principle 5: Set Limits Ahead of Time

- Do parents establish rules of behavior prior to disciplining certain behaviors on the part of the child?
- Do parents use knowledge of child development to anticipate children's behavior?
- When children engage in unacceptable behavior that is not addressed in previously established rules, do parents give a warning before instituting punishment?

Principle 6: Be Sure the Child Understands the Rules

- Are parents clear on what behavior is expected of the child and what behavior is unacceptable?

Principle 7: Prevent Rather than Punish Unacceptable Behavior

- Do parents take steps to prevent unacceptable behavior before it occurs rather than punishing it afterwards?
- Do parents remove sources of temptation from young children?
- Do parents provide adequate supervision for children?

Principle 8: Be Sure that Discipline is Warranted

- Do parents ascertain the facts of a situation before punishing children?
- Are parental expectations congruent with the child's developmental level?
- Have rules been clearly established and made clear to the child?
- Do parents attempt to determine the reason for the child's behavior and explain what is wrong when the child's intentions were good?

Principle 9: Be Sure that Discipline Is Meaningful

- Do parents make sure that the child understands the reason for punishment?
- Do parents explain how the child can correct his or her behavior?
- What form of discipline do parents use?
- Is the form of discipline used effective in modifying the child's behavior?

▶ GENERAL CONSIDERATIONS IN ASSESSING CHILDREN

- The health history and physical examination of children present golden opportunities for parent or child education.
- A health history should be obtained from a primary caretaker for young children. As children get older, they can supply much of their own history with input from caretakers as needed.
- A detailed pregnancy, birth, and neonatal history should be obtained for an infant.
- A detailed developmental history should be obtained for younger children and major developmental milestones addressed at a minimum in older children. Specific developmental tests, such as the Denver II, may be used.
- An in-depth feeding or nutritional history should be obtained with different foci for infants, children, and adolescents.
- The history of past illnesses is usually explored in more detail with children than adults. For example, one would want to know the frequency of episodes of otitis media, how they were treated, and the results for a child. Just knowing that the adult had frequent ear infections as a child is usually sufficient without additional detail.
- An immunization history is important for all clients, but particularly so for children who may not yet have initial disease protection.
- Growth should be assessed in relation to normed standards and in terms of the child's own past growth patterns.
- Respect physical modesty even in very young children. It may be helpful to allow the child to leave his or her underpants on until genitalia need to be examined then tell the child you are only going to slip them down for a moment. However, make sure that all areas of the child's skin are visually inspected at some point during the physical.
- The physical examination of a child should begin with noninvasive procedures (eg, testing EOMs) and move to more invasive ones (eg, ears and throat).
- The pace of a physical examination with a child may be slower than an adult physical due to the need for reassurance and explanation. Explanations should be offered at the level of the child's understanding. It is also wise to explain to parents what you are doing and why.
- When children need to be restrained for some parts of the physical, it may be helpful to instruct the parent or caretaker on how to restrain the child. This is less frightening for the child and also prevents parents from thinking that the nurse is using undue force to restrain a wiggly child.
- Normal physical findings will vary with the age of the child. For example, a positive Babinski is normal in a newborn, but not in an older child. Normal findings may also vary somewhat in children from different racial or ethnic backgrounds.

- Presenting signs and symptoms of illness may be different for children than adults. For example, children with pneumonia may exhibit only fever and an increased respiratory rate or may have referred abdominal pain.
- The nurse should be alert to possible evidence of child abuse or neglect and should ask caretakers about such findings.
- The nurse should also assess interactions between the child and caretaker during the history and physical examination.

▶ QUESTIONS FOR ASSESSING THE NUTRITIONAL STATUS OF CHILDREN OF SELECTED AGES

AGE GROUP	ASSESSMENT QUESTION

Infant (birth–1 year)	Is the child breast- or bottlefed?
	If breastfed:
	  How often does the child nurse?
	  How long does the child nurse?
	  Does mother alternate breasts?
	  Is mother's nutritional intake adequate?
	  Does the child seem satisfied?
	If bottlefed:
	  How often does the baby eat?
	  How much formula is consumed in 24 hours?
	  What type of formula is used? Is it iron-fortified?
	  Do parents prepare formula correctly?
	  Do parents use appropriate feeding techniques (eg, not propping the bottle)?
	  Does the infant tolerate the formula well?
	Is the infant gaining weight?
	At what point did parents introduce solids? (Recommendations are for cereal at 6 months, followed by vegetables, fruits, and meat.)
	How much solid food does the baby eat?
	Do parents use individual foods rather than less nutritious combination foods (like vegetable and beef combinations)?
	Is one new food introduced at a time? Over several days?
	Has the child started eating table food? (This usually occurs at about 9 months of age.)
	Is the child weaned from the bottle by 1 year?

AGE GROUP	ASSESSMENT QUESTION
Toddler and preschool child (2–5 years)	Which foods are the child eating? How much food is the child eating? Is the child's diet well balanced? Are finger foods and variety encouraged? Are nutritious snacks provided? Is the child given small portions initially and allowed to ask for more to enhance independence? Is the child's growth pattern normal for his or her age?
School-age child (6–12 years)	Is the child's diet well balanced? Is junk food avoided? Are snacks nutritious? How much does the child eat? Is the child overweight or underweight? Is the child's weight within normal limits for his or her age?

▶ CHILD HEALTH ASSESSMENT GUIDE

Description: This assessment guide is a basic tool for assessing the health status of children. The tool is constructed using the epidemiologic perspective of the six dimensions of health. The nurse is assisted to identify nursing diagnoses and to plan, implement, and evaluate nursing interventions to promote child health and to resolve existing health problems.

Appropriate populations: Children from birth to adolescence. Adolescents may be assessed using relevant items from this tool and from the *Health Assessment Guide—Adult Client* included in the next section of this book.

Data sources and data collection strategies: Information regarding the child's health history may be obtained in interviews with parents or other knowlegeable caretakers or from older children themselves. Other sources of information include observations by the nurse and the findings of the physical examination and screening tests. Development may be assessed using a variety of age-appropriate developmental assessment tools (eg, the Denver II for children from birth to 6 years of age). Parents may also be asked to complete a nutritional diary to provide information on child nutrition.

Use of information: Information obtained using the assessment tool is used to derive both problem-focused and wellness diagnoses. Emphasis is given to using assessment data to design interventions for promoting health and preventing illness as well as resolving existing problems. Special consideration should be given to providing parents with anticipatory guidance concerning their children's development.

▶ CHILD HEALTH ASSESSMENT GUIDE

Client's name: _____ Phone: _____
Address: _____

Assessment

Human Biology

MATURATION AND AGING

Age: _____ Date of birth: _____ Sex: _____
Race/ethnic group: _____ Birth weight and length: _____
Pattern of growth (*compared with norms and previous pattern*): _____

Accomplishment of developmental milestones (*DDST or other appropriate test*): _____

Parental knowledge of child development and its implications: _____

Significant family health history (*include genogram*): _____

PHYSIOLOGIC FUNCTION

Significant events during pregnancy: _____

Significant events during delivery: _____

Congenital defects: _____

Current acute or chronic illnesses (*describe problem, status, treatment, if any*): _____

Current signs or symptoms of physical health problems: _____

Areas of physical disability or limitation of function: _____

Significant past illnesses, injuries, hospitalizations (*what, when, outcomes*): _____

REVIEW OF SYSTEMS

Head (*headache* [how often, quality, treatment outcome], *syncope, trauma*): _____

Eyes (*vision problems, burning eyes, glasses, last eye exam, blocked tear duct, discharge, tearing, itching*): _____

Ears (*difficulty hearing, discharge, earache, frequent otitis*): _____

Mouth and throat (*sore throat, lesions, toothache, caries, last dental visit*): _____

Respiratory system (*frequent colds, nosebleeds, cough, pneumonia, asthma, shortness of breath, sinusitis, hayfever*): _____

Cardiovascular system (*heart problems, hypertension, chest pain, cyanosis* [especially when crying], *shortness of breath, murmurs, edema*): _____

Gastrointestinal system (*nausea, vomiting, diarrhea, constipation, flatulence, abdominal pain, loss of appetite, weight loss or gain, rectal pain or bleeding, quality of stool, frequency*): _____

Urinary tract (*dysuria, urinary frequency, urgency, nocturia, difficulty voiding, urinary retention, CVA pain, odor, strength of urinary stream, number of wet diapers in infant*): _____

Reproductive system (*vaginal or penile discharge, development of secondary sex characteristics, menarche, wet dreams, extent of sex education, history of STD*): _____

Musculoskeletal system (*joint pain, swelling, tremor, history of trauma, muscle weakness*): _____

Integumentary system (*eczema, diaper rash, lesions* [describe character, locale, color], *changes in skin color, itching, hair loss, discoloration or pitting of nails, clubbing of nails, birthmarks, swollen glands*): _____

Hematopoietic system (*anemia, bleeding tendencies, bruise easily, transfusions* [when, why]): _____

Immunization status: (*up-to-date for age*): _____

PHYSICAL EXAMINATION
Height, weight, head and chest circumference: _____

Vital signs (*T, P, R, B/P*): _____

General appearance (*posture, gait, deformities, hygiene*): _____

Skin (*diaper rash, eczema, acne, milia, bruises, burns, hygiene*): _____

Head and neck (*lymph nodes, face*): _____

Eyes (*ability to focus and follow objects*): _____

Ears (*ability to localize sound*): _____

Nose and sinuses: _____

Mouth and throat (*monilial patches, number of teeth, dental hygiene, caries*):
_____

Chest:
 Breast examination (*newborn engorgement, precocious puberty*): _____

 Heart (*murmurs, split heart sounds*): _____

 Lungs: _____

Abdomen: _____

Genitalia (*undescended testes, vaginal tears, discharge, imperforate anus*): ____

Musculoskeletal system (*symmetry of extremities, spina bifida, scoliosis, congenital hip dislocation*): _____

Nervous system (*cranial nerves, DTRs, temperature, kinesthetic sense, newborn reflexes*): _____

Screening test results (*PKU, T_4, hematocrit, sickle cell, serum lead, TB, urinalysis as appropriate*):_____

Environment

PHYSICAL ENVIRONMENT

Where does the client live? Is there adequate space and privacy in the home? _____

Are safety hazards present in the home? (*see Home Safety Inventory, page 21*)
_____

Are there pets in the home? (*What kind? How many? Inside or outside?*) ____

What is the neighborhood like? (*safety, pollutants, etc.*) _____
_____

PSYCHOLOGICAL ENVIRONMENT
Reactivity patterns and parental responses: _____

Parental expectations (*appropriateness*): _____

Discipline (*type, consistency, appropriateness*): _____

Parental coping skills: _____

Parent–child interactions: _____

Self-image: _____

Emotional state or mood (*usual, recent changes*): _____

Evidence of abuse or neglect: _____

Recent experience of significant loss (*death, divorce, move*): _____

Suicide ideation: _____

Level of social or parental pressure to perform: _____

SOCIAL ENVIRONMENT
Education (*grade, performance*): _____

Interaction with peers: _____

Interaction with others: _____

Cultural childrearing attitudes/practices: _____

Child care outside the home (*where, by whom, adequacy*): _____

Lifestyle

NUTRITION
Infant (*formula, breast, amount, formula preparation, feeding and burping techniques*): _____

Other age groups (*well-balanced diet, amount of "junk food," food allergies*): __

Parental knowledge of nutrition needs: _____

REST AND EXERCISE
Sleep patterns: _____

Type and amount of exercise: _____

Use of safety precautions, equipment: _____

Exposure to drugs/alcohol: _____

OTHER
Sexual activity (*frequency, use of contraceptives, condoms*): _____

Use of seat belts, other safety devices: _____

Health Care System
Use of primary prevention services (*general and dental*): _____

Source of illness care: _____

Parental knowledge of illness care and need for medical assistance: _____

Diagnosis
Biophysical Dimension

POSITIVE NURSING DIAGNOSES	NEGATIVE NURSING DIAGNOSES

Psychological Dimension

POSITIVE NURSING DIAGNOSES	NEGATIVE NURSING DIAGNOSES

Physical Dimension

POSITIVE NURSING DIAGNOSES	NEGATIVE NURSING DIAGNOSES

Social Dimension

POSITIVE NURSING DIAGNOSES	NEGATIVE NURSING DIAGNOSES

Behavioral Dimension

POSITIVE NURSING DIAGNOSES	NEGATIVE NURSING DIAGNOSES

Health System Dimension

POSITIVE NURSING DIAGNOSES	NEGATIVE NURSING DIAGNOSES

Planning

PLANNED INTERVENTIONS	OUTCOME OBJECTIVES

Implementation

INTERVENTION	RESPONSIBLE PARTY/ EXPECTED COMPLETION DATE	STATUS

Evaluation

EXPECTED OUTCOME	STATUS: MET/UNMET	SUPPORTING EVIDENCE

▶ PRIMARY PREVENTIVE INTERVENTIONS IN THE CARE OF CHILDREN

Promoting growth and development	Provide anticipatory guidance to parents.
	Assist with accomplishment of developmental tasks.
	Provide assistance with developmental concerns.
Promoting adequate nutrition	Educate parents regarding children's nutritional needs.
	Provide assistance in meeting nutritional needs.
Promoting safety	Encourage parents to provide adequate supervision of children.
	Educate parents regarding safety concerns appropriate to the child's age.
	Eliminate hazardous conditions from the environment.
	Assist parents to provide safety education appropriate to child's age and health status.
Immunization	Educate parents regarding the need for immunization and immunization schedules.
	Refer parents to immunization services.
	Educate parents about side effects of immunizations.
	Modify immunization practices or provide additional immunizations for children with special needs.
Dental care	Encourage adequate dental hygiene.
	Encourage regular dental checkups.
Support for parenting	Assist parents to develop realistic expectations of children.
	Take action to minimize parental stress.
	Assist parents to develop effective coping strategies and learn child-care skills.
	Assist parents to deal with the special needs of children with chronic illnesses or disabilities.
	Assist parents to deal with feelings of guilt, anger, and frustration engendered by a chronic or terminal condition in a child.
	Arrange respite care as needed for parents of children with chronic conditions or disabilities.

▶ NURSING INTERVENTIONS FOR COMMON HEALTH PROBLEMS IN CHILDREN

ORGAN SYSTEM	PROBLEM	INTERVENTIONS
Gastrointestinal	Spitting up	Burp baby more frequently. Keep infant upright for short time after feeding. Check size of nipple hole. Change to soy formula.
	Colic	Give small amounts of warm water. Exert gentle pressure on abdomen with infant's legs and thighs bent.
	Mild diarrhea or vomiting	Begin oral rehydration to prevent dehydration. Do not discontinue feedings. Seek medical help if condition continues or worsens.
	Constipation	Increase fluid intake. Add bulk to diet. Encourage regular toileting habits. Discourage postponing defecation. Avoid use of laxatives or enemas.
Respiratory	Mild respiratory infection	Increase fluid intake. Use a cold mist humidifier to ease breathing. Do not use Vicks Vaporub or other aromatic substances. Seek medical help for severe or persistent cough, difficulty breathing, stridor, or nasal flaring.
Integumentary	Diaper rash	Wash diapers with mild soaps and rinse thoroughly. Add ¾ cup vinegar to last rinse to remove ammonia. If using disposable diapers, use those that allow air circulation. Frequent diaper change and cleansing of diaper area.

ORGAN SYSTEM	PROBLEM	INTERVENTIONS
	Allergic dermatitis	Do not use powders or lotion in diaper area. Leave diaper area exposed when possible. Explore changes in foods or soaps. Eliminate possible causative substances. Seek medical help for severe rashes or secondary infection.
	Cradle cap	Scrub scalp with soap and soft washcloth during bath. Brush scalp with soft brush after bath. Do not use oil or lotion on scalp.
	Abrasions and lacerations	Wash with soap and water. Keep clean.
Urinary	Urinary tract infection	Seek medical assistance.
	Bedwetting	Limit fluid intake after dinner. Empty bladder before bed. Awaken child to urinate before parents go to bed. Do not make an issue of the problem. If problem is severe or continues beyond age 6, seek medical attention.
Musculoskeletal	Sprains and fractures	Perform basic first aid and immobilize injured area. Seek medical attention.
	Leg cramps	Increase calcium intake. If severe or persistent, seek medical attention.
Neurological	Headache	Give nonaspirin analgesic according to child's age and size. If severe or recurrent, seek medical attention.
	Hearing problem	Seek medical attention.
	Vision problem	Seek medical attention.

ORGAN SYSTEM	PROBLEM	INTERVENTIONS
Other	Delayed speech	Discourage older children and parents from talking for child. Encourage child to verbalize needs before meeting them. Seek medical attention for prolonged delay.
	Speech defect	Seek medical attention.
	Fever	For temperature over 102°F, give nonaspirin antipyretic. For high or persistent fever, seek medical attention.
	Suspected abuse	Refer to child protective services.
	Night terrors	Use a night light or leave bedroom door open. Use bedtime rituals of checking for "monsters" if helpful. Use a "guardian" stuffed animal to scare away monsters. Comfort the child after waking and stay until child returns to sleep. Seek assistance for persistent terrors or those related to a real traumatic event.
	Jealousy of new baby	Prepare siblings for birth of another child. Have child assist with care of newborn. Emphasize positive aspects of being older. Accept regressive behavior and do not belittle. Spend time with just the older child. Encourage friends and relatives to pay attention to older child as well as new baby.
	Sibling rivalry	Mediate arguments. Encourage children to work out own differences. Encourage compromise.

ORGAN SYSTEM	PROBLEM	INTERVENTIONS
		Give reasons for differences in privileges.
		Use role-play with older children to give insight into feelings and behaviors of others.
	Tantrums	Ignore behavior, if possible.
		Remove child to bedroom if disturbing others.
		Do not give in to child's demands.
	Bedtime	Complete bedtime rituals and put child in bed.
		Ignore crying for 15–20 minutes. If the child does not stop, see what is wrong.
		If child gets up, put him or her back to bed.
		Place several safe toys in bed with child and allow play until the child falls asleep.
	Poor self-esteem	Praise child for accomplishments.
		Correct mistakes without denigrating child.
		Help child identify and strengthen talents.
		Assist child to accept limitations.
		Seek assistance for severe depression or low self-esteem on the part of child.

SECTION IV CARE OF CLIENTS 89

▶ THE ADULT CLIENT

The essence of community health nursing is the care provided to clients to enhance their health. Nursing care for the individual client differs, of course, from that for families or groups of people. For the adult client, gender is often a factor that determines health status. Men and women experience unique health care needs, in part due to susceptibility to specific health problems, but also due to social conditions amenable to change. Community health nurses are in a unique position to assist women and men to deal with health needs and problems.

Community health nurses contribute to women's health through their roles as counselors, providers of direct care, case finders, teachers, and advocates in a health care system that too often does not accord women the same status as men. See *Nursing in the Community: Dimensions of Community Health Nursing* (Chapter 21) for an in-depth presentation of care of women.

Although a great deal of information exists about specific problems that influence men's health (eg, cardiovascular disease), very little attention has been given to the overall health needs of men. Men tend to encounter the health care system on an episodic basis, whereas women are more apt to be regular recipients of health care services. Community health nurses who may encounter men in the work setting or in the course of caring for other family members are in a position to identify unmet health care needs and to provide avenues for men's access to appropriate health care services. See *Nursing in the Community: Dimensions of Community Health Nursing* (Chapter 22) for an in-depth discussion of the care of men.

▶ DEVELOPMENTAL CHARACTERISTICS OF ADOLESCENTS AND ADULTS

11–14 years	Neurophysical	Beginning pubertal changes, gawkiness.
	Psychosocial	Importance of peer group conformity, strong identification with agemates, learning one's role in heterosexual relationships, beginning to establish an identity, more abstract thought, negative attitude to family.
15–18 years	Neurophysical	Finishing pubertal changes and adolescent growth spurt, better able to handle the "new" body.
	Psychosocial	Developing an independent identity, establishing relationships with members of the opposite sex (gay and lesbian youth

		may be coming to terms with homosexuality), adopting an adult value set, movement away from family relationships.
Early to late active adulthood	Neurophysical Psychosocial	Beginning manifestation of aging process. Developing and implementing career goals, establishing a family, becoming a productive citizen, assisting children to become independent, assisting older parents, cultivating friendships with age-mates, maintaining family relationships and learning new relationships with spouses of children and grandchildren, establishing healthy routines, learning new motor skills, mastering complex financial dealings, formulating a philosophy of life.
Late adulthood	Neurophysical	Increasing mobility limitations, sensory impairment, effects of chronic disease may manifest or become worse, decreased appetite.
	Psychosocial	Adjusting to retirement and to loss of family members and friends, keeping mentally alert, accepting help graciously, adjusting to reduced income, learning new family roles, preserving friendships, adjusting to declining strengths and stamina, maintaining social interactions, adapting activities to diminished energy, preparing for death.

► GENERAL CONSIDERATIONS IN ASSESSING MEN'S HEALTH

- Men are often unaware of the importance of specific symptoms and may not volunteer information unless specifically asked. For this reason, a thorough review of systems is particularly important in assessing the health of male clients.
- Men frequently fail to seek assistance with health problems until their ability to function is affected. Nurses who are seeing male clients, for whatever reason, should be alert to signs and symptoms of unreported health problems in order to permit early identification and intervention.
- Men may be reluctant to discuss personal or intimate issues with others, particularly female nurses. For this reason, the nurse must be particularly assiduous in explaining the purpose for soliciting this information. The

nurse should also open discussion of intimate issues in a nonjudgmental and matter-of-fact manner.
- Men may be reluctant to report information that they perceive as evidence of weakness or lack of masculinity. The nurse must approach such information in a nonjudgmental manner and assist the client to change his perceptions of what constitutes masculinity.
- Some men are reluctant to seek assistance from others, so the nurse should assess the extent of the male client's social support network as well as his ability to accept help from network members.
- Men of some cultural groups will be resistant to interactions with female nurses. Arrangements for assessment and care by a male nurse should be made, if possible.

▶ GENERAL CONSIDERATIONS IN ASSESSING WOMEN'S HEALTH

- Differences in health status indicators between men and women arise from more than reproductive differences.
- Some women may have a history of their complaints being disregarded by health care providers or incorrectly ascribed to psychological or reproductive causes. Nurses should be particularly attentive to women's assessment of their own health.
- Diagnostic criteria and interventions for many common health problems are based on research conducted with men and may not be relevant to women.
- Women may present with "atypical" symptoms for certain conditions. For example, women experiencing myocardial infarction may report neck or jaw pain rather than classic chest pain. The nurse should be alert to the possibility of such differences in assessing women's health.
- Women who are the victims of family violence may seek health care for a variety of reasons and the nurse should be alert to the possibility of abuse in women who seek care frequently. In addition, all women should be routinely asked if they are involved in abusive situations.
- Women who have responsibility for the care of others may give low priority to their own health. Nurses should pay particular attention to self-care practices by these women as well as assessing the extent of stress caused by their caretaking responsibilities.
- Women from some cultural groups will be resistant to care by male nurses. Arrangements should be made for care to be provided by female nurses when possible.

► HEALTH ASSESSMENT GUIDE—ADULT CLIENT

Description: This assessment guide is intended to assist the community health nurse to assess the health needs of adult clients and to direct the planning, implementation, and evaluation of nursing interventions to meet identified needs. The assessment component of the tool is based on the six dimensions of health in the Dimensions Model of community health nursing.

Appropriate populations: May be used with young and middle adult male and female clients. Assessment of adolescents may combine features of the *Child Health Assessment Guide* (page 76 of this handbook) with elements of this tool. Community health nurses assessing the needs of older clients should use the *Health Assessment Guide for Older Client* (page 124).

Data sources and data collection strategies: Information required for assessing adult clients is usually obtained from interviews with the client. Additional data may be obtained from health records, laboratory test results, and the observations of the nurse. For incompetent clients, data may be obtained from significant others.

Use of information: The information gleaned in the adult assessment is used by the community health nurse to make nursing diagnoses and to plan, implement, and evaluate nursing care to address clients' health needs.

▶ HEALTH ASSESSMENT GUIDE—ADULT CLIENT

Client's name: _____ Phone: _____
Address: _____

Assessment

Biophysical Dimension
MATURATION AND AGING
Age: _____ Date of birth: _____ Sex: _____
Race/ethnic group: _____
Accomplishment of adult developmental tasks: _____

Significant family health history (*include genogram*): _____

PHYSIOLOGIC FUNCTION
Current acute or chronic illnesses (*describe problem, status, treatment, if any*): _____

Current signs or symptoms of physical health problems: _____

Areas of physical disability or limitation of function: _____

Significant past illnesses, surgery, injuries, hospitalizations (*what, when, outcomes*): _____

REVIEW OF SYSTEMS
Head (*headache* [how often, quality, treatment outcome], *syncope, trauma*):

Eyes (*vision problems, burning eyes, glasses, last eye exam, blocked tear duct, discharge, tearing, itching*): _____

Ears (*difficulty hearing, discharge, earache*): _____

Mouth and throat (*sore throat, lesions, toothache, caries, last dental visit*): _____

Respiratory system (*frequent colds, nosebleeds, cough, pneumonia, asthma, shortness of breath, sinusitis, hay fever*): _____

Cardiovascular system (*heart problems, hypertension, chest pain, cyanosis, shortness of breath, murmurs, edema*): _____

Gastrointestinal system (*nausea, vomiting, diarrhea, constipation, flatulence, abdominal pain, loss of appetite, weight loss or gain, rectal pain or bleeding*): _____

Urinary tract (*dysuria, urinary frequency, urgency, nocturia, difficulty voiding, urinary retention, CVA pain*): _____

Reproductive system (*sexual satisfaction, history of STDs*): _____

- Female (*edema of labia or vulva, vaginal discharge* [color, character, odor], *use of oral or other contraceptives, pregnancies* [past or current] *and outcome, age at menarche, LMP, dysmenorrhea, irregular menses, breast discharge, breast self-exam, breast lumps, changes in breast contour, dyspareunia*): _____

- Male (*prostatitis, penile discharge* [color, character, amount], *lesions on penis, testicular self-exam, testicular pain, lumps, impotence, dysuria, scrotal swelling*): _____

Musculoskeletal system (*joint pain, swelling, tremor, history of trauma, muscle weakness*): _____

Integumentary system (*lesions* [describe character, locale, color], *changes in skin color, itching, hair loss, discoloration or pitting of nails, birthmarks, swollen glands*): _____

Neurological system (*seizures, ataxia, tics, tremors, paralysis*): _____

Hematopoietic system (*anemia, bleeding tendencies, bruise easily, transfusions* [when, why]): _____

Immunologic system (*frequent infections, HIV infection, use of immunosuppressives*): _____

Immunization status: _____

PHYSICAL EXAMINATION
Height and weight: _____
Vital signs (*T, P, R, B/P*): _____
General appearance (*posture, gait, deformities, hygiene*): _____

Skin (*include hair and nails*): _____

Head and neck (*lymph nodes, face*): _____

Eyes: _____
Ears: _____
Nose and sinuses: _____
Mouth and throat (*lips, gums, palate, pharynx, tongue, teeth*): _____

Chest:
• Breast examination: _____
• Heart: _____
• Lungs: _____
Abdomen: _____
Genitalia (*including anus and rectum, prostate in male, ovaries in female*): _____

Musculoskeletal system (*extremities, spine, joints, muscles*): _____

Nervous system (*cranial nerves, DTRs, temperature, kinesthetic sense*): _____

Results of screening and other tests: _____
_____

PSYCHOLOGICAL DIMENSION
Self-image, level of self-esteem: _____

History of mental illness: _____

Emotional mood or state (*current and recent changes*): _____

Level of orientation: _____

Coping (*strategies used, effectiveness*): _____

Recent experience of significant loss (*death, divorce, relocation, effects*): _____

Suicide ideation: _____

Communication with others (*extent, adequacy*): _____

Interpersonal relationships (*satisfaction, extent*): _____

Stress (*sources, coping skills, support*): _____

Evidence of physical or emotional abuse: _____

PHYSICAL DIMENSION

Where does the client live? Is there adequate space and privacy in the home? _____

Are safety hazards present in the home? (*See [Home Safety Inventory, page 21]*) _____

Are there pets in the home? (*What kind? How many? Inside or outside?*) ____

What is the neighborhood like? (*Describe safety, pollutants, etc.*) _____

SOCIAL DIMENSION

Education (*formal education, health knowledge, special learning needs*): ____

Income (*source, adequacy, budgeting skills*): _____

Social support network (*components, adequacy, use*): _____

Cultural practices influencing health: _____

Extent of social support for healthy behavior: _____

Religious affiliation (*importance/influence on health*): _____

Adequacy of adult role models: _____

Employment (*current and past, hazards, job change pattern*): _____

Behavioral Dimension

CONSUMPTION PATTERNS

Usual diet (*meal pattern, preferences, preparation, nutritional adequacy, special needs, cultural restrictions*): _____

Use of alcohol, tobacco, other drugs: _____

Use of caffeine: _____

Use of medications (*type, appropriateness*): _____

REST AND EXERCISE
Sleep patterns: _____

Type and amount of exercise: _____

Leisure (*type of activity, hazards posed*): _____

OTHER
Sexual activity (*frequency, use of contraceptives, condoms, sexual orientation, multiple partners, sexual practices*): _____

Use of seat belts, other safety devices: _____

Health System Dimension
Use of primary prevention services (*general and dental*): _____

Attitudes toward health and health care: _____

Usual source of health care: _____

Health care financing (*type, adequacy*): _____

Barriers to care: _____

Use of health care services (*appropriateness*): _____

Diagnosis

Biophysical Dimension

POSITIVE NURSING DIAGNOSES	NEGATIVE NURSING DIAGNOSES

Psychological Dimension

POSITIVE NURSING DIAGNOSES	NEGATIVE NURSING DIAGNOSES

Physical Dimension

POSITIVE NURSING DIAGNOSES	NEGATIVE NURSING DIAGNOSES

Social Dimension

POSITIVE NURSING DIAGNOSES	NEGATIVE NURSING DIAGNOSES

Behavioral Dimension

POSITIVE NURSING DIAGNOSES	NEGATIVE NURSING DIAGNOSES

Health System Dimension

POSITIVE NURSING DIAGNOSES	NEGATIVE NURSING DIAGNOSES

Planning

PLANNED INTERVENTIONS	OUTCOME OBJECTIVES

Implementation

INTERVENTION	RESPONSIBLE PARTY/ EXPECTED COMPLETION DATE	STATUS

Evaluation

EXPECTED OUTCOME	STATUS: MET/UNMET	SUPPORTING EVIDENCE

▶ PRENATAL CARE CHECKLIST

INTERVENTION	COMPLETED	
Biophysical Dimension	Yes	No

First Trimester
- Obtain past pregnancy history ☐ ☐
- Identify risks posed by age of mother, if any ☐ ☐
- Determine prepregnant weight, periodic weight check ☐ ☐
- Obtain medical history (eg, HIV infection, TB, diabetes) ☐ ☐
- Assess for edema ☐ ☐
- Address normal discomforts of pregnancy (eg, nausea, constipation, heartburn, urinary frequency, etc.), suggest measures for alleviation ☐ ☐
- Assess for anemia ☐ ☐
- Check blood pressure on each visit ☐ ☐
- Encourage loose fitting clothing and properly fitted shoes ☐ ☐
- Teach signs of complications ☐ ☐
- Assess for dental hygiene, problems. Encourage dental hygiene. Refer as needed for dental problems ☐ ☐
- Assess for fetal movement ☐ ☐
- Monitor existing health problems (eg, diabetes) ☐ ☐
- Assess risk for congenital problems (eg, family history, communicable disease exposure, etc.) ☐ ☐

Second Trimester
- Assess fundal height ☐ ☐
- Assess fetal heart tones ☐ ☐
- Check blood pressure regularly ☐ ☐
- Continue to monitor existing health problems ☐ ☐
- Monitor for signs of complications ☐ ☐
- Educate regarding Braxton–Hicks contractions ☐ ☐
- Assess fetal movement ☐ ☐

Third Trimester
- Assess fundal height ☐ ☐
- Assess fetal heart tones ☐ ☐
- Check blood pressure regularly ☐ ☐
- Continue to monitor existing health problems ☐ ☐
- Assess for lightening ☐ ☐
- Assess fetal position, movement ☐ ☐
- Teach signs of labor ☐ ☐
- Refer for childbirth preparation classes ☐ ☐

INTERVENTION	COMPLETED	
Psychological Dimension	Yes	No

First Trimester
- Assess feelings regarding pregnancy ☐ ☐
- Assess for emotional lability, reassure of normality ☐ ☐
- Identify preexisting mental or emotional illness, refer for care as needed ☐ ☐
- Assess for evidence of abuse, refer for assistance as needed ☐ ☐

Second Trimester
- Monitor signs of early bonding with baby ☐ ☐
- Continue to assess for possible abuse ☐ ☐

Third Trimester
- Assist client to deal with waiting, restlessness ☐ ☐
- Continue to monitor feelings regarding pregnancy ☐ ☐
- Continue to assess for possible abuse ☐ ☐

Physical Dimension

First Trimester
- Assess adequacy of living arrangements, space for new baby ☐ ☐
- Assess safety hazards in home ☐ ☐

Third Trimester
- Assist in planning sleeping arrangements for baby ☐ ☐
- Assist with reallocation of space among family members, if needed ☐ ☐

Social Dimension

First Trimester
- Assess extent of support system ☐ ☐
- Assess parental role models ☐ ☐
- Assess knowledge of child care ☐ ☐
- Assess financial status, refer for assistance as needed ☐ ☐
- Assess cultural beliefs and practices related to pregnancy ☐ ☐
- Assess relationship with father of child, other family members ☐ ☐

Second Trimester
- Begin preparation of siblings for new baby ☐ ☐

INTERVENTION	COMPLETED	
	Yes	No

Social Dimension

Third Trimester
- Assist with obtaining baby items, if needed ☐ ☐
- Encourage plans for care of other children ☐ ☐
- Assist with arranging transportation to hospital ☐ ☐
- Encourage client to explore child-care arrangements if returning to work ☐ ☐
- Continue preparation of siblings ☐ ☐
- Assist with development of new roles, reallocation of previous roles ☐ ☐
- Teach parenting skills as needed ☐ ☐

Behavioral Dimension

First Trimester
- Assess diet, educate on nutritional needs in pregnancy as needed ☐ ☐
- Refer for nutritional supplement program or counseling as needed ☐ ☐
- Encourage vitamin supplements, iron, etc. ☐ ☐
- Assess use of tobacco, alcohol, other drugs ☐ ☐
- Educate regarding effects of perinatal substance exposure as needed* ☐ ☐
- Refer for assistance with substance use/abuse, if needed ☐ ☐
- Assess for balance between rest and exercise ☐ ☐
- Encourage adequate exercise ☐ ☐
- Assess sexual activity, educate regarding alternate positions for comfort ☐ ☐
- Encourage decision on breast- or bottlefeeding ☐ ☐

Second Trimester
- Continue to encourage adequate diet, exercise, etc. ☐ ☐

Third Trimester
- Discuss plans for contraception if desired, educate as needed ☐ ☐
- Caution against sexual activity late in trimester ☐ ☐

Health System Dimension

First Trimester
- Refer for prenatal care if not yet obtained ☐ ☐

INTERVENTION	COMPLETED	
Health System Dimension	*Yes*	*No*
Second Trimester • Encourage continued prenatal care	☐	☐
Third Trimester • Encourage continued prenatal care	☐	☐

---

* See table of fetal, neonatal, and developmental effects of perinatal psychoactive substance exposure on page 225 of this handbook.

▶ POSTPARTUM/NEWBORN VISIT INTERVENTION CHECKLIST

BIOPHYSICAL DIMENSION

- Check blood pressure ☐ ☐
- Check fundal height ☐ ☐
- Check lochia ☐ ☐
- Examine breasts for cracks or fissures ☐ ☐
- Check episiotomy ☐ ☐
- Assess infant growth pattern (height, weight, head/chest circumference) ☐ ☐
- Assess infant hygiene ☐ ☐
- Conduct physical examination of newborn ☐ ☐
- Reassure mother regarding normal newborn variations, molding, etc. ☐ ☐
- Assess bowel and bladder function (mother and newborn) ☐ ☐
- Assess infant developmental level ☐ ☐

PSYCHOLOGICAL DIMENSION

- Assess for postpartum depression ☐ ☐
- Assess maternal–infant bonding ☐ ☐
- Assess parental expectations of infant ☐ ☐
- Assess expectations of self as parent ☐ ☐
- Encourage client to verbalize regarding labor and delivery experience ☐ ☐

PHYSICAL DIMENSION

- Assess sleeping arrangements for infant ☐ ☐
- Assess adequacy of living conditions ☐ ☐

SOCIAL DIMENSION

- Assess impact of infant on family ☐ ☐
- Assess sibling response to newborn ☐ ☐
- Assess financial impact of infant ☐ ☐
- Encourage time alone with other children, if any ☐ ☐
- Provide assistance with sibling rivalry as needed ☐ ☐
- Assess ability to cope with role changes ☐ ☐
- Assist with plans to return to work, as needed (eg, child-care arrangements) ☐ ☐
- Assess extent of support system and client's ability to accept help ☐ ☐

- Assess cultural beliefs and practices related to post-partum/newborn period ☐ ☐
- Assess relationship with extended family ☐ ☐
- Assess relationship with father of child ☐ ☐

BEHAVIORAL DIMENSION

- Educate regarding postpartum/breastfeeding diet ☐ ☐
- Educate regarding infant nutrition ☐ ☐
- Encourage breastfeeding ☐ ☐
- Observe feeding technique (breast or bottle), educate as needed ☐ ☐
- Discourage early introduction of foods for infant ☐ ☐
- Refer for food supplement programs, if needed ☐ ☐
- Encourage regular exercise ☐ ☐
- Educate regarding resumption of sexual activity ☐ ☐
- Assess need for contraceptives, educate or refer as needed ☐ ☐
- Discuss effects of alcohol, drugs on breast milk ☐ ☐
- Discuss effects of smoking on newborn, if mother smokes ☐ ☐
- Observe child care techniques, educate as needed ☐ ☐
- Educate regarding infant safety practices ☐ ☐
- Assess infant wake/sleep patterns ☐ ☐
- Encourage regular breast self-examination ☐ ☐

HEALTH SYSTEM DIMENSION

- Refer for postpartum check if appointment not yet made ☐ ☐
- Educate regarding infant immunizations ☐ ☐
- Educate regarding minor illness care ☐ ☐
- Refer for well child services, immunizations ☐ ☐
- Refer for contraceptive services as needed ☐ ☐

▶ TECHNIQUES FOR TEACHING BREAST SELF-EXAMINATION (BSE)

Materials needed:
- BSE pamphlets (available from American Cancer Society)
- BSE video and equipment (if available)
- Flip chart or poster showing technique for BSE
- Folded towel
- Breast model(s)
- BSE contract for each participant

Learning objectives: At the conclusion of the presentation, participants should be able to:
- Verbalize the importance of regular BSE
- Verbalize appropriate timing of BSE in the menstrual cycle
- Demonstrate correct BSE technique

Teaching strategies:
- Begin with figures on the incidence of breast cancer as a focusing event. Personalize the statistics by saying "Two of the women in this room will develop breast cancer in the next 5 years." Modify your statement, as needed, to reflect breast cancer incidence relative to the size of the audience.
- Present risk factors for breast cancer. Determine how many members of the audience have identified risk factors.
- Discuss risk factor modification strategies.
- Focus discussion on BSE with a statement such as, "When eliminating risk factors doesn't work, it's important to discover breast cancer as early as possible."
- Present the advantages of early detection of breast cancer through BSE, manual breast examination, and mammography.
- Discuss timing of BSE during the menstrual cycle for women who are still menstruating.
- Demonstrate BSE techniques.
  > Discuss visual inspection of breasts and what women should be looking for (changes in contour, marked assymetry, dimpling, etc.).
  > Demonstrate visual inspection with arms at sides, arms extended overhead, and hands on hips and pressing down.
  > Demonstrate palpation of breast with a towel under the shoulder on the side to be examined and hand behind head and using a spiral motion with the flat of the fingers to spiral from the tail of the breast inward to the nipple, moving the fingers only in small increments until the entire breast has been examined.

- > Demonstrate squeezing breast to check for discharge.
- > Demonstrate palpation of the axillary area for enlarged lymph nodes.
- Have participants palpate the breast model to feel what they are palpating for.
- Have participants verbalize and demonstrate visual breast inspection.
- Have participants verbalize and demonstrate correct BSE palpation techniques on self or breast model.
- Provide a brief summary of BSE timing and technique.
- Close presentation by having participants make a signed contract with themselves to perform monthly BSE.

▶ TECHNIQUES FOR TEACHING TESTICULAR SELF-EXAMINATION (TSE)

Materials needed:
- TSE pamphlets (available from American Cancer Society)
- TSE video and equipment (if available)
- Flip chart or poster showing technique for TSE
- Model(s) of scrotum and testes
- TSE contract for each participant

Learning objectives: At the conclusion of the presentation, participants should be able to:
- Verbalize the importance of regular TSE
- Verbalize the best time for conducting TSE
- Demonstrate correct TSE technique

Teaching strategies:
- As a focusing event, give participants a self-test on risk factors for testicular cancer.
- Discuss testicular cancer risk factors.
- Discuss the advantages of early detection of testicular tumors.
- Discuss showering as the best time to conduct TSE when scrotum is relaxed.
- Demonstrate TSE technique on model.
  > Demonstrate isolation of testicle within scrotum and use of fingers of both hands to palpate for lumps on front and sides.
  > Show placement of epididymis on back of testicle and reassure that it is not a testicular lump.
- Have participants verbalize and demonstrate correct TSE technique on model.
- Summarize importance and technique for TSE.
- Close presentation by having participants make a signed contract with themselves to perform monthly TSE.

▶ THE OLDER CLIENT

Increased longevity and a lower birth rate in the United States have contributed to significant growth in the elderly as a percentage of the population. Although life expectancy continues to increase, the quality of life for the elderly is often questionable. In working with the older adult, community health nurses must be concerned with quality of life as well as longevity.

Aging is a normal human phenomenon surrounded by myths, including beliefs that aging is a time of tranquillity, is synonymous with senility, and is marked by reduced productivity and resistance to change. Another myth presents aging as a uniform process with similar outcomes for all. For many older adults, however, aging is a time of increased problems and decreased resources for dealing with them. Senility is not an inevitable consequence of aging, and many older persons retain their mental faculties and remain productive well beyond the ninth and tenth decades of life. Aging brings unique effects to each person, and the outcomes of aging may differ widely from one individual to another.

Much can be done by the community health nurse to enhance the health status of the elderly population, improve their quality of life, and decrease the health care costs associated with the needs of this population. See *Nursing in the Community: Dimensions of Community Health Nursing* (Chapter 23) for an in-depth presentation of care of older clients.

▶ COMMON PHYSICAL CHANGES OF AGING AND THEIR IMPLICATIONS FOR HEALTH

SYSTEM AFFECTED	CHANGES NOTED	IMPLICATIONS FOR HEALTH
Integumentary system		
Skin	Decreased turgor, sclerosis, and loss of subcutaneous fat, leading to wrinkles	Lowered self-esteem
	Increased pigmentation, cherry angiomas	
	Cool to touch, dry	Itching, risk of injury, insomnia
	Decreased perspiration	Hyperthermia, heat stroke

SYSTEM AFFECTED	CHANGES NOTED	IMPLICATIONS FOR HEALTH
Hair	Thins, decreased pigmentation	Lowered self-esteem
Nails	Thickened, ridges, decreased rate of growth	Difficulty trimming nails, potential for injury
Cardiovascular system	Less efficient pump action and lower cardiac reserves	Decreased physical ability and fatigue with exertion
	Thickening of vessel walls, replacement of muscle fiber with collagen	Elevated blood pressure, varicosities, venous stasis, pressure sores
	Pulse pressure up to 100	
	Arrythmias and murmurs	
	Dilated abdominal aorta	
Respiratory system	Decreased elasticity of alveolar sacs, skeletal changes of chest	Decreased gas exchange, decreased physical ability
	Slower mucous transport, decreased cough strength, dysphagia	Increased potential for infection or aspiration
	Postnasal drip	
Gastrointestinal system	Wearing down of teeth	Difficulty chewing
	Decreased saliva production	Dry mouth, difficulty digesting starches
	Loss of taste buds	Decreased appetite, malnutrition
	Muscle atrophy of cheeks, tongue, etc.	Difficulty chewing, slower to eat
	Thinned esophageal wall	Feeling of fullness/heartburn after meals
	Decreased peristalsis	Constipation
	Decreased hydrochloric acid and stomach enzyme production	Pernicious anemia, frequent eructation

SYSTEM AFFECTED	CHANGES NOTED	IMPLICATIONS FOR HEALTH
	Decreased lip size, sagging abdomen	Change in self-concept
	Atrophied gums	Poorly fitting dentures, difficulty chewing, potential for mouth ulcers, loss of remaining teeth
	Decreased bowel sounds	Potential for misdiagnosis
	Fissures in tongue	
	Increased or decreased liver size (2–3 cm below costal border)	Potential for misdiagnosis
Urinary system	Decreased number of nephrons and ability to concentrate urine	Nocturia, increased risk of falls
Reproductive system		
Female	Atrophied ovaries, uterus	Ovarian cysts
	Atrophy of external genitalia, pendulous breasts, small flat nipple, decreased pubic hair	Lowered self-esteem
	Scant vaginal secretions	Dyspareunia
	Vaginal mucosa thin and friable	
Male	Decreased size of penis and testes, decreased pubic hair, pendulous scrotum	Lowered self-esteem
	Enlarged prostate	Difficulty urinating, incontinence
Musculoskeletal system	Decreased muscle size and tone	Decreased physical ability
	Decreased range of motion in joints affecting gait, posture, balance, and flexibility	Increased risk of falls, decreased mobility

SYSTEM AFFECTED	CHANGES NOTED	IMPLICATIONS FOR HEALTH
	Kyphosis	Lowered self-esteem
	Joint instability	Increased risk of falls, injury
	Straight thoracic spine	
	Breakdown of chondrocytes in joint cartilage	Osteoarthritis, joint pain, reduced ability for activities of daily living
	Osteoporosis	Increased risk of fracture
Neurological system	Diminished hearing, vision, touch, increased reaction time	Increased risk of injury, social isolation
	Diminished pupil size, peripheral vision, adaptation, accommodation	
	Diminished sense of smell, taste	Decreased appetite, malnutrition
	Decreased balance	Increased risk of injury
	Decreased pain sensation	Increased risk of injury
	Decreased ability to problem solve	Difficulty adjusting to new situations
	Diminished deep tendon reflexes	
	Decreased sphincter tone	Incontinence (fecal or urinary)
	Diminished short-term memory	Forgetfulness
Endocrine system		
Thyroid	Irregular, fibrous changes	
Female	Decreased estrogen and progesterone production	Osteoporosis, menopause
Male	Decreased testosterone production	Fatigue, weight loss, decreased libido, impotence, lowered self-esteem, depression

► CHANGES IN NORMAL LABORATORY VALUES IN OLDER CLIENTS

TEST	YOUNG ADULT NORMAL	OLDER ADULT NORMAL
Urine		
Protein	0–5 mg/100 mL	Up to 30 mg/100 mL
Glucose	0–15 mg/100 mL	Declines slightly
Specific gravity	1.032	1.024
Blood		
Hemoglobin	*Men:* 13–18 g/100 mL	*Men:* 10–17 g/100 mL
	Women: 12–16 g/100 mL	*Women:* No change
Leukocytes	4300–10,800/mm^3	3100–9000/mm^3
Lymphocytes	*T:* 500–2500/mm^3	Declines
	B: 50–200/mm^3	Declines
Platelets		Increased platelet release factors, decreased granular consistency, no change in absolute number
Beta-globulin	2.3–3.5 g/100 mL	Increases slightly
Sodium	135–145 mEq/L	134–147 mEq/L
Potassium	3.5–5.5 mEq/L	Increases slightly
Blood urea nitrogen (BUN)	*Men:* 10–25 mg/100 mL *Women:* 8–20 mg/100 mL	69 mg/100 mL
Creatinine	0.6–1.5 mg/100 mL	*Men:* 1.9 mg/100 mL *Women:* No change
Glucose tolerance (GTT)	1 h: 160–170 mg/100 mL 2 h: 115–125 mg/100 mL 3 h: 70–110 mg/100 mL	Rises faster in first 2 h, then declines more slowly
Triglycerides	40–150 mg/100 mL	20–200 mg/100 mL
Cholesterol	120–220 mg/100 mL	*Men:* Decreases after age 50 *Women:* Increases from age 50–70, then decreases
Thyroxine (T$_4$)	4.5–13.5 μg/100 mL	Declines by 25%
Triiodothyronine (T$_3$)	90–220 mg/100 mL	Declines by 25%
Thyroid-stimulating hormone (TSH)	13–39 IU/L	Increases 8–10 IU/L

TEST	YOUNG ADULT NORMAL	OLDER ADULT NORMAL
Creatinine kinase (CK)	17–48 U/L	Increases slightly
Lactate dehydrogenase (LDH)	45–90 U/L	Increases slightly

Source: Gardner, B. C. (1989). Guide to changing lab values in elders. *Geriatric Nursing, 10*(3), 144–145.

▶ GENERAL CONSIDERATIONS IN ASSESSING OLDER ADULTS

- The normal effects of aging must be differentiated from pathology.
- Normal effects of aging are constantly being redefined.
- Normal laboratory values and other findings may differ between younger and older adults.
- Older clients may exhibit atypical signs and symptoms of illness.
- Older clients may exhibit a decreased tolerance for stress.
- Strengths that result from an older client's life experiences may provide a basis for health interventions.
- Loss is a persistent theme in the lives of older adults.
- Older clients usually exhibit multiple health problems that have complex interactions.
- Older clients may underreport symptoms of illness.
- Older clients may have multiple, nonspecific complaints that require explication.
- Older clients may have difficulty communicating their health needs.

▶ FUNCTIONAL HEALTH STATUS INVENTORY

Description: This inventory is intended to assist the community health nurse to assess clients' functional abilities. It addresses function in relation to basic, instrumental, and advanced activities of daily living

Appropriate populations: Adult clients. May be particularly useful for home health clients and those with chronic or disabling conditions. May also be used to assess the functional status of clients with dementia or other mental and emotional health problems.

Data sources and data collection strategies: Data may be collected via interviews with clients or significant others or through observation of client abilities.

Use of information: Information gleaned from the inventory can be used to identify areas where nursing intervention is needed for clients to function more effectively. Data are also used to tailor nursing interventions for other health problems to clients' capabilities.

▶ FUNCTIONAL HEALTH STATUS INVENTORY

ACTIVITY	STATUS	
Basic Activities of Daily Living	Yes	No

Feeding
- Can the client feed him- or herself? ☐ ☐
- Does the client have difficulty chewing? ☐ ☐
- Does the client have difficulty swallowing? ☐ ☐

Bathing
- Can the client get into or out of the bathtub or shower? ☐ ☐
- Can the client manipulate soap and washcloth? ☐ ☐
- Can the client wash his or her hair without assistance? ☐ ☐
- Can the client effectively dry all body parts? ☐ ☐

Dressing
- Can the client remember what articles of clothing should be put on first? ☐ ☐
- Can the client dress him- or herself? ☐ ☐
- Can the client bend and reach to put on shoes and stockings? ☐ ☐
- Can the client manipulate buttons and zippers? ☐ ☐
- Are modifications in clothing required to facilitate dressing (eg, front opening dresses)? ☐ ☐
- Is arm and shoulder movement adequate to put on and remove sleeves? ☐ ☐
- Can the client comb his or her hair? ☐ ☐
- Can the client apply makeup if desired? ☐ ☐

Toileting
- Is the client mobile enough to reach the bathroom? ☐ ☐
- Is there urgency that may lead to incontinence? ☐ ☐
- Can the client remove clothing in order to urinate or defecate? ☐ ☐
- Can the client position him- or herself on or in front of the toilet? ☐ ☐
- Can the client lift from a sitting position on the toilet? ☐ ☐
- Is the client able to effectively clean him- or herself after urinating or defecating? ☐ ☐
- Can the client replace clothing after urinating or defecating? ☐ ☐

Transfer
- Is the client able to get from a lying to a sitting position unassisted? ☐ ☐

ACTIVITY	STATUS	
Basic Activities of Daily Living	Yes	No
• Is the client able to stand from a sitting position without support or assistance?	☐	☐
• Is the client able to sit or lie down without help?	☐	☐
Instrumental Activities of Daily Living	Yes	No

Shopping
- Is the client able to transport him- or herself to shopping facilities? ☐ ☐
- Can the client navigate within a shopping facility? ☐ ☐
- Can the client lift products from shelves? ☐ ☐
- Can the client effectively handle money? ☐ ☐
- Can the client carry purchases from store to car and from car to home? ☐ ☐
- Is the client able to store purchases appropriately? ☐ ☐

Laundry
- Can the client collect dirty clothes for washing? ☐ ☐
- Is the client able to sort clothes to be washed from those to be dry cleaned? ☐ ☐
- Can the client sort clothes by color? ☐ ☐
- Can the client access laundry facilities? ☐ ☐
- Can the client manipulate containers of soap, bleach, etc.? ☐ ☐
- Can the client lift wet clothing from washer to dryer? ☐ ☐
- Is the client able to hang or fold clean clothes as needed? ☐ ☐
- Can the client put clean clothing in closets or drawers? ☐ ☐

Cooking
- Is the client capable of planning well-balanced meals? ☐ ☐
- Can the client safely operate kitchen utensils and appliances (eg, stove, can opener)? ☐ ☐
- Can the client reach dishes, pots, and pans needed for cooking and serving food? ☐ ☐
- Can the client clean vegetables and fruits, chop foods, etc.? ☐ ☐
- Is the client able to carry prepared foods to the table? ☐ ☐

Housekeeping
- Can the client identify the need for housecleaning chores (eg, when the tub needs to be cleaned)? ☐ ☐
- Is the client able to do light housekeeping (eg, dusting, vacuuming, cleaning toilet)? ☐ ☐
- Is the client able to do heavy chores (eg, scrub floors, wash windows)? ☐ ☐
- Is the client able to do yard maintenance, if needed? ☐ ☐

ACTIVITY	STATUS	
Instrumental Activities of Daily Living	Yes	No
Taking Medication		
• Can the client remember to take medications as directed?	☐	☐
• Is the client able to open medication bottles?	☐	☐
• Can the client swallow oral medication, administer injections, etc., as needed?	☐	☐
Managing Money		
• Can the client effectively budget his or her income?	☐	☐
• Is the client able to write checks?	☐	☐
• Can the client balance a checking account?	☐	☐
• Can the client remember to pay bills when due and record payment?	☐	☐
Advanced Activities of Daily Living	Yes	No
Social Activity		
• Does the client have a group of people with whom he or she can socialize?	☐	☐
• Is the client able to transport him- or herself to social events?	☐	☐
• Can the client see and hear well enough to interact socially with others?	☐	☐
• Does the client tire too easily to engage in social activities?	☐	☐
• Is social interaction impeded by fears of incontinence or embarrassment over financial difficulties?	☐	☐
Occupation		
• Can the client carry out occupational responsibilities as needed?	☐	☐
Recreation		
• Does the client have the physical strength and mobility to engage in desired recreational pursuits?	☐	☐
• Does the client have the financial resources to engage in desired recreational pursuits?	☐	☐
• Does the client have a group of people with whom to engage in recreation?	☐	☐
• Does the client have access to recreational activities (eg, transportation)?	☐	☐

▶ COGNITIVE FUNCTION ASSESSMENT GUIDE

Description: This tool is intended to assist the community health nurse to assess clients' cognitive function.

Appropriate populations: Adult clients who may be at risk for diminished cognitive function, particularly those who have evidence of dementia. May also be used with depressed clients or those with other mental or emotional illness. Assessment data should be interpreted within the client's cultural context.

Data sources and data collection strategies: Data may be collected via interviews with clients or significant others or through observation of client abilities.

Use of information: Information gleaned from the assessment is used to develop nursing interventions to improve clients' cognitive status when possible and to design nursing interventions for other health problems that are congruent with client's cognitive abilities.

▶ COGNITIVE FUNCTION ASSESSMENT GUIDE

ASSESSMENT AREA	STATUS	
	Yes	No

Attention Span
- Does the client focus on a single activity to completion? ☐ ☐
- Does the client move from activity to activity without completing any? ☐ ☐

Concentration
- Is the client able to answer questions without wandering from the topic? ☐ ☐
- Does the client ignore irrelevant stimuli while focusing on a task? ☐ ☐
- Is the client easily distracted from a subject or task by external stimuli? ☐ ☐

Intelligence
- Does the client understand directions and explanations given in everyday language? ☐ ☐
- Is the client able to perform basic mathematical calculations? ☐ ☐

Judgment
- Does the client engage in action appropriate to the situation? ☐ ☐
- Are client behaviors based on an awareness of environmental conditions and possible consequences of action? ☐ ☐
- Are the client's plans and goals realistic? ☐ ☐
- Can the client effectively budget income? ☐ ☐
- Is the client safe driving a car? ☐ ☐

Learning Ability
- Is the client able to retain instructions for a new activity? ☐ ☐
- Can the client recall information provided? ☐ ☐
- Is the client able to correctly demonstrate new skills? ☐ ☐

Memory
- Is the client able to remember and describe recent events in some detail? ☐ ☐
- Is the client able to describe events from the past in some detail? ☐ ☐

ASSESSMENT AREA	STATUS	
	Yes	No

Orientation
- Can the client identify him- or herself by name? ☐ ☐
- Is the client aware of where he or she is? ☐ ☐
- Does the client recognize the identity and function of those around them? ☐ ☐
- Does the client know what day and time it is? ☐ ☐
- Is the client able to separate past, present, and future? ☐ ☐

Perception
- Are the client's responses appropriate to the situation? ☐ ☐
- Does the client exhibit evidence of hallucinations or illusions? ☐ ☐
- Are explanations of events consistent with the events themselves? ☐ ☐
- Can the client reproduce simple figures? ☐ ☐

Problem Solving
- Is the client able to recognize problems that need resolution? ☐ ☐
- Can the client envision alternative solutions to a given problem? ☐ ☐
- Can the client weigh alternative solutions and select one appropriate to the situation? ☐ ☐
- Can the client describe activities needed to implement the solution? ☐ ☐

Psychomotor Ability
- Does the client exhibit repetitive movements that interfere with function? ☐ ☐

Reaction Time
- Does the client take an unusually long time to respond to questions or perform motor activities? ☐ ☐
- Does the client respond to questions before the question is completed? ☐ ☐

Social Intactness
- Are the client's interactions with others appropriate to the situation? ☐ ☐
- Is the client able to describe behaviors appropriate and inappropriate to a given situation? ☐ ☐

▶ HEALTH ASSESSMENT GUIDE FOR THE OLDER CLIENT

Description: This tool is designed to use in assessing the health status of older clients. It is framed in terms of the nursing process and directs assessment, diagnosis, planning, implementation, and evaluation of community health nursing care for older adults. The assessment component of the tool reflects the six dimensions of health included in the Dimensions Model.

Appropriate populations: All older adult clients. May also be used with groups of older adults to identify problems common in population groups.

Data sources and data collection strategies: Interviews with or observations of older clients and physical examination may be used to obtain most of the assessment data included in the tool. For older clients who are cognitively impaired, information may be obtained in interviews with significant others. Medical and other records may also be a source of assessment data.

Use of information: Information obtained through use of the assessment tool is used to plan individualized nursing interventions to meet the health needs of the older adult client.

▶ HEALTH ASSESSMENT GUIDE FOR THE OLDER CLIENT

Client's name: _____ Phone: _____
Address: _____

Assessment

Biophysical Dimension

PHYSIOLOGIC FUNCTION

Perceptions of personal health: _____
_____

REVIEW OF SYSTEMS (INCLUDE EFFECTS OF AGING)

Eyes (*visual impairment, use of glasses*): _____
_____

Ears (*hearing impairment, use of hearing aid*): _____
_____

Mouth and throat (*dentures* [*fit, use*], *dry mouth, bleeding gums*): _____

Integumentary (*skin integrity, fragility, dryness, itching, lesions, bruises, bleeding, skin color changes, hair distribution, thickened nails; hair, nail, and skin care practices; temperature of extremities, decreased perspiration*): _____
_____

Respiratory (*shortness of breath with exertion, cyanosis, emphysema, cough*): ___
_____

Cardiovascular (*history of heart disease, palpitations, hypertension, effect of activity on heart rate, edema, fatigue, orthostatic hypotension, varicosities, venous ulcers*): _____

Gastrointestinal (*flatulence, constipation, heartburn, rectal bleeding, incontinence, dysphagia, appetite, ability to chew*): _____

Musculoskeletal (*mobility, joint swelling, pain, use of cane or other device, history of fractures, kyphosis*): _____

Neurological (*seizures, ataxia, tics, tremors, paralysis, diminished sense of smell, touch, heat sensation, taste, numbness or tingling*): _____

Reproductive (*decreased libido*): _____
• Male (*difficulty in achieving erection, prostatitis, impotence*): _____

- Female (*onset of menopause, last Pap smear, mammogram, breast self-exam*): __
  _____

Urinary (*frequency, urgency, incontinence, color, odor, nocturia*): _____

Immunologic (*frequent infection, HIV infection, use of immunosuppressives*): __

Hematopoietic (*anemia, epistaxis, bleeding tendencies*): _____

Existence of acute and chronic health problems (*diagnosis, status, treatment, effects*): _____

Functional abilities related to:
 Bathing: _____

 Dressing: _____

 Toileting: _____

 Mobility: _____

 Eating: _____

 Bowel and bladder function: _____

 Communicating: _____

Immunization status (*tetanus, diphtheria, pneumonia, influenza*): _____

PSYCHOLOGICAL DIMENSION
Mental status/orientation: _____

Changes in self-image due to aging, retirement: _____

Adjustment to retirement: _____

Coping abilities: _____

History of mental illness: _____

Provision for privacy: _____

Loss of loved ones: _____

Life satisfaction: _____

Preparation for death: _____

Evidence of depression: _____

Evidence of abuse or neglect: _____

PHYSICAL DIMENSION
Safety hazards in home (*See Home Safety Inventory, page 21*): _____

Presence of safety features in home: _____

Availability of resources in neighborhood: _____

Neighborhood safety: _____

Driving: _____

Home maintenance and repair: _____

Pets: _____

Adequacy of heating, lighting, ventilation: _____

SOCIAL DIMENSION
Social interaction and support network: _____

Income (*source, adequacy, ability to budget*): _____

Relationships with family: _____

Education level: _____

Religion and importance in client's life: _____

Ethnicity and influence on client's health: _____

Possibility of institutionalization and client response: _____

Current employment: _____

Previous occupation:_____

Behavioral Dimension
CONSUMPTION PATTERNS
Nutrition (*adequacy for needs, special needs, appetite, meal pattern, food preferences and modes of preparation, food supplements, food storage, shopping practices*): _____

Use of alcohol or other drugs: _____

Use of medications (*type, appropriateness, effectiveness*): _____

Exercise: _____

Sleep patterns: _____

LEISURE ACTIVITIES
Preferred leisure pursuits: _____

Opportunity for leisure activities: _____

SEXUALITY
Opportunity for intimacy: _____

Alternative modes of meeting sexual needs:_____

INDEPENDENCE
Ability to care for self: _____

Ability to make independent decisions: _____

Health System Dimension
Source of health care: _____

Health care financing (*Medicare, insurance*): _____

Use of health care services: _____

Barriers to obtaining health care: _____

Diagnosis

Biophysical Dimension

POSITIVE NURSING DIAGNOSES	NEGATIVE NURSING DIAGNOSES

Psychological Dimension

POSITIVE NURSING DIAGNOSES	NEGATIVE NURSING DIAGNOSES

Physical Dimension

POSITIVE NURSING DIAGNOSES	NEGATIVE NURSING DIAGNOSES

Social Dimension

POSITIVE NURSING DIAGNOSES	NEGATIVE NURSING DIAGNOSES

Behavioral Dimension

POSITIVE NURSING DIAGNOSES	NEGATIVE NURSING DIAGNOSES

Health System Dimension

POSITIVE NURSING DIAGNOSES	NEGATIVE NURSING DIAGNOSES

Planning

PLANNED INTERVENTIONS	OUTCOME OBJECTIVES

Implementation

INTERVENTION	RESPONSIBLE PARTY/ EXPECTED COMPLETION DATE	STATUS

Evaluation

EXPECTED OUTCOME	STATUS: MET/UNMET	SUPPORTING EVIDENCE

▶ PRIMARY PREVENTION STRATEGIES FOR OLDER ADULTS

AREA OF CONCERN	PRIMARY PREVENTION STRATEGIES
Nutrition	Educate clients regarding nutritional needs.
	Promote caloric intake adequate to meet energy needs.
	Encourage well-balanced diet high in nutrient content (especially calcium, iron, vitamins A and C, riboflavin and thiamine, and fiber).
	Discourage participation in food fads.
	Maintain hydration.
Hygiene	Bathe periodically with mild soaps.
	Use lotion to prevent drying of skin.
	Keep hands out of water or wear gloves.
	Maintain oral hygiene with good toothbrush.
	Maintain hydration to prevent dry mouth.
	Brush and comb hair daily.
	Shampoo weekly with mild soap and condition monthly.
Safety	Wear hat to protect scalp from sunburn.
	Wear properly fitted clothes and shoes.
	Use electric blanket rather than hot water bottles.
	Provide adequate lighting, especially on stairs.
	Use a nightlight at night and keep a flashlight handy.
	Place furniture to prevent falls.
	Keep electrical cords short and tack along baseboards.
	Eliminate throw rugs, if possible, or use nonskid type.
	Install tub rails and other safety fixtures.
	Discourage use of space heaters, kerosene stoves, and similar devices.
	Install smoke alarms.
	Notify police and fire personnel of older person in home.
	Promote adequate and safe heating and ventilation of home.
	Provide door and window locks and keep car locked.
	Do not admit strangers to home.
	Ride with others or use a bus rather than drive if senses are impaired.
	Use care in crossing streets.
	Promote family coping abilities and relieve stress to prevent abuse of older persons

AREA OF CONCERN	PRIMARY PREVENTION STRATEGIES
Immunization	Encourage adequate immunization for diphtheria and tetanus.
	Provide annual influenza immunization.
	Provide pneumonia vaccine.
Rest and exercise	Encourage moderate exercise on a regular basis.
	Arrange activities to accommodate rest periods as needed.
Maintaining independence	Provide support services that allow clients to live independently, if possible.
	Encourage family members to foster independence.
	Encourage client participation in health care planning.
	Advocate for client independence as needed.
Life resolution and preparation for death	Encourage reminiscence.
	Assist client to discuss death with family members.
	Assist client to put affairs on order.

▶ SECONDARY PREVENTION FOR COMMON PROBLEMS IN OLDER ADULTS

CLIENT PROBLEM	SECONDARY PREVENTIVE STRATEGIES
Skin breakdown	Inspect extremities regularly for lesions.
	Keep lesions clean and dry.
	Eliminate pressure by frequent changes of position.
	Refer for treatment as needed.
Constipation	Encourage fluid and fiber intake.
	Discourage ignoring urge to defecate.
	Encourage regular exercise.
	Encourage regular bowel habits.
	Use mild laxatives as needed, but discourage overuse.
	Administer enemas as needed; discourage overuse.
	Administer bulk products or stool softeners as indicated.
Urinary incontinence	Refer for urological consult.
	Encourage frequent voiding.
	Teach Kegel exercises.
	Assist with bladder training.
	Encourage use of sanitary pads, panty liners, etc., with frequent changes of such aids.
	Keep skin clean and dry; change clothing and linen as needed.

CLIENT PROBLEM	SECONDARY PREVENTIVE STRATEGIES
	Offer bedpan or urinal frequently or assist to bedside commode at frequent intervals.
Sensory loss	Provide adequate lighting.
	Keep eyeglasses clean and hearing aids functional.
	Eliminate safety hazards.
	Use large-print books or materials.
	Use multisensory approaches to communication and teaching.
	Avoid using colors that make discrimination difficult.
	Speak clearly and slowly, at a lower pitch.
	Eliminate background noise.
	Assist clients to obtain voice enhancers for phone.
	Use additional herbs and spices, but use with discretion.
	Purchase small amounts of perishable foods.
	Check pilot lights on gas appliances frequently.
	Encourage the use of smoke detectors.
Mobility limitation	Provide assistance with ambulation, transfer, etc.
	Assist clients to obtain equipment such as walkers and wheelchairs.
	Install ramps, tub rails, etc., as needed.
	Promote access to public facilities for older persons.
	Assist clients to find sources of transportation.
	Make referrals for assistance with personal care or instrumental activities.
Pain	Plan activities for times when pain is controlled.
	Encourage warm soaks.
	Encourage adequate rest and exercise to prevent mobility limitations.
Confusion	Apply principles of reality orientation.
Depression	Accept feelings and reflect on their normality; encourage client to ventilate feelings.
	Refer for counseling as needed.
Social isolation	Compensate for sensory loss; enhance communication abilities.
	Improve mobility; provide access to transportation.
	Assist client to obtain adequate financial resources.
	Refer client to new support systems.
	Assist client to deal with grief over loss of loved ones.
Abuse or neglect	Assist caretakers to develop positive coping strategies.
	Assist families to obtain respite care or day care for older members.

CLIENT PROBLEM	SECONDARY PREVENTIVE STRATEGIES
	Refer families for counseling as needed.
	Arrange placement in temporary shelter.
	Assist families in making other arrangements for safe care of older clients.
Alcohol abuse	Identify problem drinking by older clients.
	Refer for therapy, Alcoholics Anonymous or Al-Anon as appropriate.
	Observe for toxic effects of alcohol ingestion.
	Maintain hydration and nutrition.
Inadequate financial resources	Refer for financial assistance.
	Assist with budgeting and priority allocation.
	Educate for less expensive means of meeting needs.
	Function as an advocate as needed.

▶ PRINCIPLES OF REALITY ORIENTATION

- Limit stimulation, provide a calm environment
- Maintain a regular daily routine
- Speak concisely, phrase questions and answers in clear, easily understood language
- Gain the client's attention and speak directly to him or her
- Provide clear instructions or directions
- Break tasks down to simple component parts and give direction in sequence, one step at a time
- Provide frequent reminders of date, time, and place
- Keep client focused and prevent rambling speech
- Be firm but gentle in directing client
- Be sincere
- Be consistent

▶ THE FAMILY CLIENT

The family, although changeable and as unique as its individual members, is the most enduring social institution. The family has been the basis for procreation, socialization, and continuation of cultures since the beginning of human history. As social norms have evolved over the centuries, many have predicted that the family would cease to exist as a social institution. Yet the family unit continues as a viable social structure and, thus, is an important consideration for community health nurses.

Families can take many forms, including nuclear conjugal families, extended families, single-parent families, stepfamilies, cohabiting families, homosexual families, and communal families. Community health nurses contribute to the growth and health of the community and society through the care they provide to family groups. See *Nursing in the Community: Dimensions of Community Health Nursing* (Chapter 18) for an in-depth discussion of care of the family client.

▶ STAGES OF FAMILY DEVELOPMENT

STAGE	TIME FRAME	DEVELOPMENTAL TASKS
I Beginning family	"Marriage" to birth of first child	1. Establish mutually satisfying marriage 2. Relate to kin network 3. Family planning
II Early childbearing	Birth of first child plus 30 months	1. Establish stable family unit 2. Reconcile conflict in developmental tasks 3. Facilitate developmental tasks of members
III Family with preschool children	Oldest child 2–5 years of age	1. Integrate second or third child 2. Socialize children 3. Begin separation from children

STAGE	TIME FRAME	DEVELOPMENTAL TASKS
IV Family with school-age children	Oldest child 6–13 years of age	1. Separate from children to a greater degree 2. Foster education and socialization 3. Maintain marriage
V Family with teenage children	Oldest child 13–20 years of age	1. Maintain marriage 2. Develop new communication channels 3. Maintain standards
VI Launching center family	From time first child leaves to time last child leaves	1. Promote independence 2. Integrate spouses of children into family 3. Restore marital relationship 4. Develop outside interests 5. Assist aging parents
VII Family of middle years	From time last child leaves to retirement	1. Cultivate leisure activities 2. Provide healthful environment 3. Sustain satisfying relationships with parents and children
VIII Family in retirement and old age	Retirement to death	1. Maintain satisfying living arrangements 2. Adjust to decreased income 3. Adjust to loss of spouse

Source: Friedman, M. M. (1998). *Family nursing: Research, theory and practice* (4th ed.). Stamford, CT: Appleton & Lange.

▶ HEALTH ASSESSMENT AND INTERVENTION PLANNING GUIDE—FAMILY CLIENT

Description: This tool incorporates the Dimensions Model to assess the health needs of families as the recipients of care by community health nurses and to plan, implement, and evaluate that care. The assessment portion of the tool addresses factors in each of the six dimensions of health that may influence the health of the family.

Appropriate populations: Appropriate to all types of families (eg, nuclear or extended families, blended families). May also be used with families from a variety of cultural groups.

Data sources and data collection strategies: The primary source of data will be interviews with family members and observations made by the community health nurse. The nurse may also obtain information from other persons to whom the family is well known. The nurse should, however, be sure to obtain the consent of the family before seeking information from outside sources such as health care providers, teachers, and so on.

Use of information: Information obtained in the family assessment is used to make nursing diagnoses related to family health status and to identify problems that require nursing intervention. Family problems for which intervention may be required may be more or less directly related to health. For example, a referral for financial assistance is much less directly related to health status than providing services such as immunizations. Based on the nursing diagnoses derived from assessment data, the community health nurse plans, implements, and evaluates interventions specifically designed to fit the family's circumstances, taking into account their strengths and ameliorating areas of difficulty.

▶ HEALTH ASSESSMENT AND INTERVENTION PLANNING GUIDE— FAMILY CLIENT

Assessment

Family surname(s): _____ Phone: _____
Address: _____

Biophysical Dimension

NAME	AGE	SEX	PHYSICAL HEALTH STATUS

MATURATION AND AGING
Individual family members' developmental tasks met? _____

Effects of individual development on family health: _____

Significant past health problems of family members: _____

PHYSIOLOGIC FUNCTION
Treatment for family members' current health problems (*type, effects, source*): _____

Significant family history of hereditary conditions: _____

Immunization status of family members: _____

PSYCHOLOGICAL DIMENSION
Family strengths and weaknesses: _____

Family communication (*typical patterns, effectiveness, purposes, tone, rules*): __

Family stage of development: _____

Status of developmental tasks of this and previous stages: _____

Extent of emotional support for family members: _____

Coping strategies used (*type, effectiveness*): _____

Discipline (*type, source, consistency, appropriateness*): _____

History of mental illness in family members: _____

Family roles:

ROLE	PERFORMED BY	ADEQUACY	ROLE MODEL
Leader			
Child care			
Sexual			
Breadwinner			
Confidant			
Disciplinarian			
Homemaker			
Repairperson			
Financial manager			

Presence of role conflict or role overload: _____

Family goals (*congruence with individual and societal goals*): _____

Sources of stress for family members: _____

PHYSICAL DIMENSION
Family home (*location, adequacy for family size*): _____

Safety hazards present in home: _____

Neighborhood (*safety, services and facilities available, pollutants*): _____

SOCIAL DIMENSION
Religious affiliations of family members and their influence on health: ____

Family cultural affiliations and influences on health: _____

Family income (*source, adequacy, effectiveness of management*): _____

Education level of family members: _____

External resources available to family: _____

OCCUPATION

FAMILY MEMBER	OCCUPATION	EMPLOYER

Occupational health hazards for family members: _____

Behavioral Dimension
CONSUMPTION PATTERNS
Family dietary patterns (*amount, food preferences, preparation, adequacy, special needs*): _____

Use of other substances (*tobacco, alcohol, other drugs*): _____

Use of prescription and nonprescription medications: _____

Rest and exercise patterns: _____

LEISURE ACTIVITY
Typical leisure activities of family members: _____

Health hazards posed by family leisure pursuits: _____

Use of recreational activities to enhance family cohesion: _____

OTHER BEHAVIORS
Use of safety devices and practices: _____

Family planning (*need for, type, effectiveness*): _____
_____

Health System Dimension
Family attitudes toward health: _____
_____

Family response toward illness: _____
_____

Use of folk remedies and self-care practices: _____
_____

Usual source of health care: _____
_____

Means of financing health care: _____
_____

Barriers to obtaining health care: _____
_____

Diagnosis
Biophysical Dimension

POSITIVE NURSING DIAGNOSES	NEGATIVE NURSING DIAGNOSES

Psychological Dimension

POSITIVE NURSING DIAGNOSES	NEGATIVE NURSING DIAGNOSES

Physical Dimension

POSITIVE NURSING DIAGNOSES	NEGATIVE NURSING DIAGNOSES

Social Dimension

POSITIVE NURSING DIAGNOSES	NEGATIVE NURSING DIAGNOSES

Behavioral Dimension

POSITIVE NURSING DIAGNOSES	NEGATIVE NURSING DIAGNOSES

Health System Dimension

POSITIVE NURSING DIAGNOSES	NEGATIVE NURSING DIAGNOSES

Planning

PLANNED INTERVENTIONS	OUTCOME OBJECTIVES

Implementation

INTERVENTION	RESPONSIBLE PARTY/ EXPECTED COMPLETION DATE	STATUS

Evaluation

EXPECTED OUTCOME	STATUS: MET/UNMET	SUPPORTING EVIDENCE

▶ FAMILY CRISIS ASSESSMENT GUIDE

Description: This tool is designed to assess both the potential for family crisis and the effects of factors in each of the six dimensions of health in a crisis situation.

Appropriate populations: Families in crisis or those at risk for crisis.

Data sources and data collection strategies: The primary source of data will be interviews with family members and personal observations made by the community health nurse. The nurse may also obtain information from other persons to whom the family is well known. The nurse should, however, be sure to obtain the consent of the family before seeking information from outside sources such as health care providers, teachers, and so on.

Use of information: Information obtained in the family crisis assessment is used to identify the potential for family crisis or to assess the factors influencing the family's response to an actual crisis. Information about potential crises can be used to initiate primary preventive measures designed to avert crisis. In the case of an actual crisis, assessment information will assist the community health nurse to design interventions that capitalize on family strengths while assisting the family to effectively resolve the crisis.

▶ FAMILY CRISIS ASSESSMENT GUIDE

BIOPHYSICAL DIMENSION	YES	NO
Are family members entering transitional periods in personal development (eg, adolescence)?	☐	☐
Is the family entering a transition period in its development (eg, birth of a child)?	☐	☐
Does the health status of one or more family members increase the risk of crisis?	☐	☐
Will existing health problems impede the family's ability to deal effectively with a crisis?	☐	☐

PSYCHOLOGICAL DIMENSION

Does the family have effective coping skills?	☐	☐
Is the family capable of working together to resolve a crisis?	☐	☐
Do family members exhibit closeness?	☐	☐
Do family members exhibit insight into the potential for crisis in their situation?	☐	☐
Do family members exhibit insight into factors affecting a crisis situation?	☐	☐
Is the family "crisis-prone?"	☐	☐
Does the family have a history of successfully resolving past crises?	☐	☐
Does mental or emotional illness in the family increase the risk of crisis?	☐	☐
Has mental or emotional illness in a family member precipitated a crisis?	☐	☐
Are any family members seriously depressed?	☐	☐
Is there a risk for suicide for any family member?	☐	☐
Is there a risk for homicide in the family?	☐	☐

PHYSICAL DIMENSION

Do family living conditions increase the risk of crisis?	☐	☐

SOCIAL DIMENSION

Does the family have a strong social support network?	☐	☐
Do family interactions give rise to the potential for crisis?	☐	☐
Does the family's financial situation contribute to the risk of crisis?	☐	☐
Does the family's financial situation impede their ability to respond effectively to crisis?	☐	☐

	YES	NO
Does stress in the occupational setting give rise to the potential for family crisis?	☐	☐
Does the family have access to emotional, financial, or material support from others?	☐	☐

BEHAVIORAL DIMENSION

	YES	NO
Do any family members abuse psychoactive substances?	☐	☐
Has substance abuse precipitated a family crisis?	☐	☐
Does substance abuse impede the family's ability to respond effectively to crisis?	☐	☐
Do family members have access to recreational and leisure activities to decrease stress?	☐	☐
Do family members engage in recreational and leisure activities that promote cohesion?	☐	☐

HEALTH SYSTEM DIMENSION

	YES	NO
Does the family have health insurance coverage to deal with a health care crisis?	☐	☐
Is the family knowledgeable about resources for dealing with factors such as substance abuse or terminal illness that may precipitate crises?	☐	☐
Have extensive medical bills precipitated a family crisis?	☐	☐

▶ POPULATION GROUPS

When a community health nurse provides care to aggregates, the recipient of care—the client—may be an entire community or a subgroup within a community. Community health nurses working with population groups identify client needs and direct action to meet those needs.

Community assessment has been identified as one of the core public health functions of community health nurses. An accurate assessment is the basis of any community health endeavor and is essential to planning any program designed to meet health-related needs. Without a clear picture of the health needs of the population, health care providers have no way to determine whether current programs meet health needs or how to plan programs that will.

See *Nursing in the Community: Dimensions of Community Health Nursing* (Chapter 19) for an in-depth presentation of care of population groups.

▶ SOURCES OF COMMUNITY ASSESSMENT DATA

TYPE OF DATA	SOURCE	EXAMPLE
Quantitative	Census figures	Age composition of population
		Racial composition of population
	Local agencies	Child abuse incidence figures from child protective services
		Diabetes admissions from hospitals
		Immunization levels from schools
	Community surveys	Frequency of health services use
		Common health problems
	Observation	Number and types of educational institutions
		Number and types of recreational opportunities
	Newspaper reports	Incidence of homicide
		Incidence of motor vehicle fatalities
	Telephone book	Number and types of health care providers
		Number and types of churches
Qualitative	Community surveys	Attitudes toward health
		Attitudes toward specific health issues

TYPE OF DATA	SOURCE	EXAMPLE
	Key informant interviews	Perceptions of community health needs
	Resident interviews	Perceptions of health needs
	Observation	Quality of housing
	Participant observation	Barriers to health care for handicapped individuals

► HEALTH ASSESSMENT AND INTERVENTION PLANNING GUIDE— COMMUNITY CLIENT

Description: This tool is designed to assist the community health nurse to identify health problems exhibited by communities or population groups. The assessment component of the tool is based on the six dimensions of health addressed in the Dimensions Model, and the community health nurse is prompted to obtain information on factors in the biophysical, psychological, physical, social, behavioral, and health system dimensions as they affect community health status. The tool also provides guidance for the development of community nursing diagnoses and for planning, implementing, and evaluating interventions to address identified community health problems.

Appropriate populations: Geopolitical communities or jurisdictions. May also be applied, with modification, to specific target populations within or across geopolitical jurisdictions. See *Nursing in the Community: Dimensions of Community Health Nursing* (Appendix J).

Data sources and data collection strategies: See *Sources of Community Assessment Data* on page 148 of this handbook for a list of possible sources of data for community assessment and the types of data that might be available from each source. Data collection strategies usually need to be quite varied and may include review of records of community government agencies (including those from local health departments), health care institutions and agencies, schools, chamber of commerce, and so on, as well as interviews with key individuals in these and other organizations. Other strategies for obtaining community assessment information include interviews or surveys of community residents, review of local historical materials, participation in the activities of local groups, review of the telephone directory and other local directories listing service agencies, review of area maps, and walking or driving through the community to make personal observations. Generally speaking, the magnitude and complexity of a community assessment suggest that data collection is more effectively handled by a group of people rather than a single community health nurse. The community health nurse, however, may initiate the assessment process and coordinate data collection activities, in addition to obtaining information him- or herself. The community health nurse should also be actively involved in analysis, interpretation, and dissemination of community assessment findings and in planning programs to address community health problems.

Use of information: Information gleaned from the community assessment is used to develop community nursing diagnoses that describe health risks/problems in the community and the resources available within the community for dealing with these risks and problems. From the community nursing diagnoses, planning groups can begin to design community-based interventions to address health concerns. Again, this requires active participation of multiple individuals and agencies in the community and is not an activity that the community health nurse is likely to perform as an independent individual. As noted earlier, however, community health nurses should be actively involved in the planning, implementation, and evaluation of community health programs.

▶ HEALTH INTERVENTION PLANNING GUIDE—COMMUNITY CLIENT

Assessment

Human Biology

Births (*annual rate, extent of illegitimacy, abortion*): _____

Composition of population:

AGE	TOTAL	MALE	FEMALE	WHITE	AFRICAN AMERICAN	LATINO	ASIAN	NATIVE AMERICAN
<1 year								
1–5 years								
6–12 years								
13–20 years								
21–30 years								
31–50 years								
51–65 years								
66–80 years								
>80 years								

Mortality rates (*overall, age-specific, cause-specific*): _____

Morbidity:

DISEASE	INCIDENCE	PREVALENCE

How do morbidity and mortality rates compare with previous years? With state and national rates? _____

What is the immunization status of the population? Are there special immunization considerations? _____

Psychological Dimension
Future prospects for the community: _____

Significant events in community history: _____

Interaction of groups within the community (*racial tension, etc.*): _____

Protective services (*adequacy, local crime rate, insurance rates*): _____

Communication network (*media, informal channels, links to outside world*): ___

Sources of stress in the community: _____

Extent of mental illness in the community: _____

Physical Dimension
Community location (*boundaries, urban/rural*): _____

Size and density: _____

Prominent topographical features: _____

Housing (*type, condition, adequacy, number of persons per dwelling, sanitation*):

Safety hazards present in the environment: _____

Source of community water supply: _____

Sewage and waste disposal: _____

Nuisance factors: _____

Potential for disaster: _____

Social Dimension

Government (*type, effectiveness, community officials*): _____

Unofficial leaders (*significant informants*): _____

Political affiliations of community members: _____

Status of minority groups (*influence, length of residence*): _____

Languages spoken by community members: _____

Community income levels (*poverty, coverage by assistance programs*): _____

Education (*prevailing levels, attitudes, facilities*): _____

Religion (*major affiliations, programs and services, influence on health*): _____

Culture (*affiliation, influence on health*): _____

Employment level: _____

Transportation (*type, availability, cost, adequacy*): _____

Shopping facilities (*type, availability, cost, use*): _____

Social services (*type, availability, adequacy, use*): _____

Primary occupations of community members: _____

Major employers (*occupational health programs*): _____

Occupational hazards: _____

Behavioral Dimension

CONSUMPTION PATTERNS

Nutrition (*general levels, preferences, preparation, special needs, prevalence of anemia, obesity*): _____

Alcohol (*consumption patterns, extent of abuse*): _____

Drug use (*licit and illicit*): _____

Smoking (*extent, cessation program availability*): _____

Exercise (*extent, type, opportunity*): _____

LEISURE ACTIVITIES

Primary leisure activities of community members: _____

Recreational facilities (*availability, adequacy, cost*): _____

Health hazards posed by recreation: _____

OTHER BEHAVIORS

Use of safety devices: _____

Contraceptive use: _____

Health System Dimension

Community attitudes toward health and health services (*definitions, support of services*): _____

Health services and resources (*type, availability, cost, adequacy, utilization*): __

Prenatal care (*availability, use*): _____

Emergency services (*availability, adequacy*): _____

Health education services (*availability, adequacy*): _____

Health care financing (*extent of insurance coverage, Medicaid, Medicare, tax support*): _____

Diagnosis

Biophysical Dimension

COMMUNITY HEALTH NEED/RISK	NEED–SERVICE MATCH/MISMATCH

Psychological Dimension

COMMUNITY HEALTH NEED/RISK	NEED–SERVICE MATCH/MISMATCH

Physical Dimension

COMMUNITY HEALTH NEED/RISK	NEED–SERVICE MATCH/MISMATCH

Social Dimension

COMMUNITY HEALTH NEED/RISK	NEED–SERVICE MATCH/MISMATCH

Behavioral Dimension

COMMUNITY HEALTH NEED/RISK	NEED–SERVICE MATCH/MISMATCH

Health System Dimension

COMMUNITY HEALTH NEED/RISK	NEED–SERVICE MATCH/MISMATCH

Planning

PLANNED INTERVENTIONS	OUTCOME OBJECTIVES

Implementation

EXPECTED OUTCOME	STATUS: MET/UNMET	SUPPORTING EVIDENCE

Evaluation

INTERVENTION	RESPONSIBLE PARTY/ EXPECTED COMPLETION DATE	STATUS

SECTION V

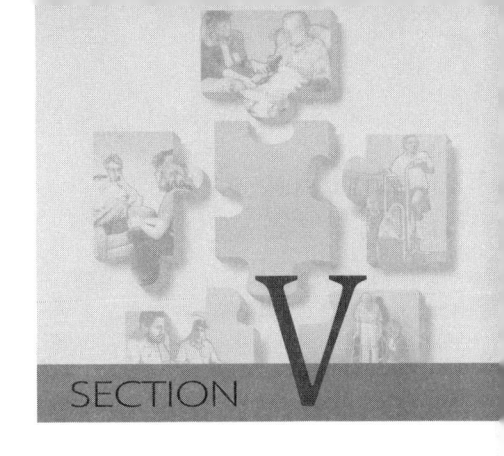

PRACTICE SETTINGS

▶ SCHOOL SETTINGS

Education and health have a reciprocal relationship. Health factors influence one's ability to learn. Education affects one's ability to engage in healthful behaviors. This reciprocal relationship makes the school setting an ideal place to provide health care.

Community health nurses working in school settings have a threefold concern for the health of schoolchildren. First, the health of schoolchildren influences the health of the community-at-large. Second, health promotion and illness prevention efforts directed at youngsters will improve their health as adults. Third, healthy children learn better and can take greater advantage of the educational opportunities provided to them. Nursing care in school settings is also directed toward the health of other members of the school population, including teachers, administrators, and staff.

Community health nurses may perform a variety of roles in the school setting, including consultant, director, educator, supervisor, coordinator, school nurse practitioner, school community nurse, and school nurse. See *Nursing in the Community: Dimensions of Community Health Nursing* (Chapter 25) for an in-depth presentation of care of clients in the school setting.

▶ ACUTE AND CHRONIC PHYSICAL HEALTH PROBLEMS ENCOUNTERED IN THE SCHOOL SETTING

ORGAN SYSTEM AFFECTED	CONDITIONS ENCOUNTERED
Cardiovascular system	Heart murmurs, hypertension
Central nervous system	Mental retardation, blindness, deafness, attention deficit hyperactivity disorder, learning disability, seizure disorder, meningitis, cerebral palsy
Endocrine system	Diabetes mellitus, thyroid disorders
Gastrointestinal system	Encopresis, hepatitis, diarrhea, dental caries, constipation, peptic and duodenal ulcer
Genitourinary/reproductive system	Sexually transmitted diseases, urinary tract infection, enuresis, dysmenorrhea, pregnancy
Hematopoietic system	Anemia, hemophilia, leukemia, sickle cell disease, lead poisoning
Immunologic system	AIDS and related opportunistic infections
Integumentary system	Acne, eczema, impetigo, lice, scabies, dermatitis, tinea corporis
Musculoskeletal system	Arthritis, sprains, fractures, scoliosis, Legg–Calve–Perthes disease
Respiratory system	Upper and lower respiratory infections, strep throat, influenza, asthma, hay fever, pertussis, diphtheria, pneumonia
Other diseases	Measles, mumps, rubella, scarlet fever, chickenpox, infectious mononucleosis, otitis media, otitis externa, conjunctivitis, Lyme disease, cancer, hepatitis

▶ CONDITIONS TYPICALLY WARRANTING EXCLUSION FROM SCHOOL AND GUIDELINES FOR READMISSION

CONDITION	READMISSION GUIDELINES
Bacterial conjunctivitis	After acute symptoms subside
Chickenpox	5 days after eruption of the first vesicles or after lesions are dried
Diphtheria	Until negative cultures of nose and throat are obtained at least 24 hours after discontinuing antibiotics

CONDITION	READMISSION GUIDELINES
Hepatitis A	1 week after onset of jaundice
Impetigo (staphylococcal)	24 hours after treatment is initiated
Influenza	After acute symptoms subside
Measles	4 days after onset of the rash
Meningococcal meningitis	24 hours after chemotherapy is initiated or when the child is sufficiently recovered
Mononucleosis, infectious	After acute symptoms subside; delay resumption of strenuous physical activity until spleen is nonpalpable
Mumps	9 days after onset of swelling
Pediculosis	24 hours after application of an effective pediculocide
Pneumonia, pneumococcal and *Mycoplasma*	48 hours after initiation of antibiotics or when child is sufficiently recovered
Pertussis	After 5 days of antibiotic therapy or when child is sufficiently recovered
Respiratory disease (viral) and upper respiratory infection	After acute symptoms subside
Rubella	7 days after onset of the rash
Scabies	24 hours after treatment
Streptococcus (strep, throat, scarlet fever, impetigo)	24 hours after treatment is initiated or when child is sufficiently recovered
Tinea corporis	Excluded only from gym, swimming pool, or other activities where exposure of other individuals may occur; activities resume after treatment is completed

► HEALTH ASSESSMENT IN THE SCHOOL SETTING

Description: This tool is designed to assist the community health nurse to apply the Dimensions Model to the care of groups of clients in the school setting. It is intended to assess the health status of school populations rather than individual students or school personnel. Assistance in directing care of individuals in the school setting can be found in other tools included in this handbook. (See the *Child Health Assessment Guide* on page 76 or the *Health Assessment Guide—Adult Client* on page 93).

Appropriate populations: The tool provided here can be used with any school population from the preschool or day care setting to college. It can also be used with different cultural groups within school settings.

Data sources and data collection strategies: Sources of data used in the assessment of school health status will include reviews of school records; interviews with school personnel, parents, and students; interviews with representatives of other community agencies and organizations that interact with the school; and personal observations by the nurse. Surveys of students, staff, families, and community members may also be used to obtain information on health in the school setting.

Use of information: Information gleaned from the assessment of the health status of the school population will be used for a variety of purposes. One major use of the data is in the design of school health programs to meet identified health needs. Information may also be used to plan a health education curriculum in areas that address identified needs. Finally, information on the health status of school populations may be used to direct community planning efforts designed to improve the health status of the broader community or to enhance the effectiveness of school–community interaction with respect to health.

▶ HEALTH ASSESSMENT IN THE SCHOOL SETTING

Biophysical Dimension
Age, sex, and racial/ethnic composition of the school population: _____

Extent of developmental delays among students: _____

Specific developmental considerations: _____

Presence of handicapping conditions: _____

Incidence of communicable disease *(students and staff)*: _____

Incidence and prevalence of chronic disease *(students and staff)*: _____

Prevalence of genetic predisposition to disease: _____

Immunization status: _____

Psychological Dimension
Organization of the school day *(appropriateness to needs, effects on health)*: __

Aesthetic quality of environment: _____

Relationships among students *(quality, appropriateness of adult monitoring)*: _____

Teacher–student relations *(quality, extent)*: _____

Teacher–teacher relations: _____

Discipline *(type, extent, appropriateness, consistency, fairness)*: _____

Grading practices *(consistency, fairness)*: _____

Parent–school relations *(quality, extent)*: _____

Sources of stress in the school environment: _____

Physical Dimension
Traffic patterns around the school: _____

Safety hazards in the neighborhood: _____

Use of pesticides and other poisons in the neighborhood: _____

Pollutants in the area of the school: _____

Fire or safety hazards in the school environment: _____

Use of toxic chemicals in labs, art classes, cleaning, and maintenance: _____

Use of hazardous equipment in home economics or "shop" classes: _____

Broken glass in recreational areas: _____

Play equipment in poor repair: _____

Hard surfaces below play equipment: _____

Animals in the school environment: _____

Plant allergens or poisons in the school environment: _____

Adequacy of heating, lighting, cooling: _____

Noise levels: _____

Food sanitation practices: _____

Toilet facilities (*adequacy, state of repair*): _____

Cleaning of shower facilities: _____

Isolation facilities for students with communicable diseases: _____

Facilities and access for handicapped students or staff: _____

Social Dimension

Community attitudes toward education and toward school: _____

Community support of school program: _____

Crime in neighborhood (*extent, effect on school and student health*): _____

Funding (*source, extent, adequacy, priorities*): _____

Home environment of students: _____

Availability of before- and after-school care: _____

Socioeconomic status of students, staff: _____

Presence of intergroup conflicts: _____

Cultural background of staff, students: _____

Education level of families and extent of health knowledge: _____

Extent of homelessness among students: _____

Behavioral Dimension
CONSUMPTION PATTERNS
Quality of school meal programs: _____

Student/staff nutritional levels: _____

Special nutritional needs (*students or staff*): _____

Nutrition knowledge (*extent among students, staff, parents*): _____

Extent of alcohol or drug use by students, staff, family members: _____

Extent of smoking by students, staff, family members: _____

Medication use (*types, dispensing policies*): _____

EXERCISE AND LEISURE ACTIVITIES
Rest and exercise patterns of school population: _____

Recreational opportunities (*type, age-appropriateness*): _____

Use of appropriate safety equipment: _____

OTHER
Sexual activity by students (*extent, use of contraceptives, use of condoms and other barrier devices*): _____

Use of safety devices (*seat belts*): _____

Health System Dimension

Health care services offered by school: _____

Availability of other health care services: _____

Use of health care services by school population: _____

Financing of health care services *(source, adequacy)*: _____

Emphasis placed on health in school curriculum: _____

Support of school health program by health care professionals in the community: _____

School and community attitudes toward health and health care: _____

Diagnosis

Biophysical Dimension

POPULATION HEALTH NEED/ RISK	NEED–SERVICE MATCH/MISMATCH

Psychological Dimension

POPULATION HEALTH NEED/ RISK	NEED–SERVICE MATCH/MISMATCH

Physical Dimension

POPULATION HEALTH NEED/ RISK	NEED–SERVICE MATCH/MISMATCH

Social Dimension

POPULATION HEALTH NEED/ RISK	NEED–SERVICE MATCH/MISMATCH

Behavioral Dimension

POPULATION HEALTH NEED/ RISK	NEED–SERVICE MATCH/MISMATCH

Health System Dimension

POPULATION HEALTH NEED/ RISK	NEED–SERVICE MATCH/MISMATCH

Planning

PLANNED INTERVENTIONS	OUTCOME OBJECTIVES

Implementation

INTERVENTION	RESPONSIBLE PARTY/ EXPECTED COMPLETION DATE	STATUS

Evaluation

EXPECTED OUTCOME	STATUS: MET/UNMET	SUPPORTING EVIDENCE

▶ PRIMARY PREVENTION IN THE SCHOOL SETTING AND RELATED COMMUNITY HEALTH NURSING RESPONSIBILITIES

AREA OF EMPHASIS	COMMUNITY HEATH NURSING RESPONSIBILITIES
Immunization	Refer for immunization services as needed.
	Provide routine immunizations.
	Suggest additional immunizations as warranted by circumstances (eg, an epidemic of hepatitis A).
Safety	Report safety hazards to appropriate authorities.
	Provide safety education.
	Collaborate with others to eliminate safety hazards in the community.
School exclusion	Determine need for exclusion from school.
	Explain need for exclusion to parents.
	Refer child for treatment of condition, if needed.
	Educate students and parents on preventing the spread of communicable diseases.
	Follow up on students excluded from school to ensure appropriate care.
Health education	Participate in designing health education curricula.
	Provide consultation to teachers on health education topics.
	Provide in-service for teachers related to health education.
	Teach health education in the classroom.
	Arrange for other health educational experiences (eg, field trips or guest speakers).
	Arrange or provide health education for families.
Food and nutrition	Provide consultation on menu planning.
	Educate students and families regarding nutrition.
Self-image	Provide a role model for teachers and others in positive interactions with students.
	Provide consultation to teachers on activities to enhance student's self-esteem.
	Function as an advocate for students who have poor self-esteem.
Coping skills	Provide a role model for students and staff for effective problem-solving skills.
	Provide counseling regarding problem-solving skills.

AREA OF EMPHASIS	COMMUNITY HEATH NURSING RESPONSIBILITIES
Interpersonal skills	Reinforce use of appropriate coping skills. Educate students and staff on stress and coping. Provide a role model for students and staff for effective interpersonal skills. Educate students, staff, and parents on group dynamics and communication skills.

▶ SECONDARY PREVENTION IN THE SCHOOL SETTING AND RELATED COMMUNITY HEALTH NURSING RESPONSIBILITIES

AREA OF EMPHASIS	RELATED COMMUNITY HEALTH NURSING RESPONSIBILITIES
Screening	Conduct screening tests or arrange for screening by others. Train volunteers in screening procedures. Interpret screening test results. Notify parents of screening test results. Make referrals for further tests or treatment as needed. Follow up on referrals to determine outcomes and to ensure appropriate care for identified conditions.
Referral	Refer students and families for health care and other services as needed. Refer other school personnel for needed services.
Counseling	Assist students, staff, or families to make informed health decisions. Counsel students, staff, or families regarding personal problems. Assist students, staff, or families to engage in problem solving.
Treatment	Provide first aid for illness or injury. Dispense medications prescribed for acute or chronic illnesses. Perform special treatments or procedures warranted by identified conditions. Teach others to perform special treatments or procedures. Monitor therapeutic effects and side effects of medications and other treatments.

▶ TERTIARY PREVENTION IN THE SCHOOL SETTING AND RELATED COMMUNITY HEALTH NURSING RESPONSIBILITIES

AREA OF EMPHASIS	RELATED COMMUNITY HEALTH NURSING RESPONSIBILITIES
Preventing recurrence of acute conditions	Eliminate risk factors for the condition. Teach students, staff, or parents how to prevent recurrence of problems. Make referrals that can assist in eliminating risk factors.
Preventing complications of and promoting adjustment to chronic and handicapping conditions	Assist parents with finding sources of financial aid to deal with chronic and handicapping conditions. Facilitate meeting special nutritional needs. Assist with meeting special needs for transportation and facilities. Provide for special equipment needs. Promote psychological well-being. Assist students, families, and staff to deal with the eventuality of death in terminal illnesses. Refer for counseling as needed. Function as an advocate as needed.
Preventing adverse effects of learning disabilities	Provide consultation for teachers in dealing with student's learning disabilities. Participate in the design of individualized learning programs for students with learning disabilities. Function as an advocate for the learnin disabled child as needed. Serve as a role model in positively reinforcing the child's accomplishments.

▶ WORK SETTINGS

Because most adults in the United States are employed, the work setting is an important place for promoting the health of the general population. Although the work environment contributes to a wide variety of health problems, it also provides opportunities to influence a major segment of the population regarding personal health behaviors.

Over the years, employers have come to appreciate that healthy employees are more productive and that it is in the employer's interest to promote and maintain employee health. Moreover, the escalating cost of health insurance makes health promotion increasingly cost-effective. One way that some companies have chosen to decrease health-related costs is to provide on-site care for employees.

Given their knowledge of community health principles, community health nurses are uniquely prepared to meet the health needs of the working population. Their many and varied roles in an occupational setting include promoting the health of the employee population, preventing illness and injury, providing preemployment assessment of prospective employees, conducting periodic screening tests, monitoring the work environment for health hazards, providing first aid for injuries, treating existing health problems, and planning, implementing, and evaluating occupational health programs. See *Nursing in the Community: Dimensions of Community Health Nursing* (Chapter 26) for in-depth presentation of care of clients in the work setting.

▶ HEALTH HAZARDS IN SELECTED OCCUPATIONAL SETTINGS

HAZARD	OCCUPATIONAL SOURCES	HEALTH EFFECTS
Asbestos	Construction, renovation	Lung cancer, respiratory effects
Communicable disease	Ranching, dairy or poultry farming, health care, child care, veterinary medicine, meat packing, sanitation	Respiratory or gastrointestinal effects
Cumulative trauma/ vibration	Secretarial work, word processing, meat packing, some construction, work involving repetitive movement	Cumulative trauma disorders (CTDs)

HAZARD	OCCUPATIONAL SOURCES	HEALTH EFFECTS
Dust	Agriculture, graineries	Respiratory effects, asthma
Electrical hazard	Utilities, work involving electronics, construction	Electrocution
Extreme weather exposure	Utilities, construction, trucking, agriculture, road maintenance	Hypo- or hyperthermia, sunburn
Fire	Fire personnel, chemical manufacture, food preparation	Burns, asphyxiation
Heat	Agriculture, mining, manufacturing	Heat stroke, reproductive effects, hearing loss
Heavy metals		
Antimony	Iron works, red dye manufacture	Irritation, cardiovascular and lung effects
Arsenic	Photographic equipment manufacture	Lung and lymphatic cancer, dermatitis
Cadmium	Soldering, battery manufacture, fuses paint manufacture, painting, nuclear reactors	Lung cancer, prostatic cancer, renal system effects
Chromium	Steel manufacture, chrome plating, dye and paint manufacture	Lung cancer, skin ulcers, lung irradiation
Lead	Soldering; dispensing leaded gas; cable cutting and splicing; painting, casting, or melting lead; radiator repair; welding; grinding or sanding lead-painted surfaces; battery manufacture; paper hanging; construction; foundries; plumbing	Kidney, blood, and nervous system effects
Mercury	Metal foil and leaf application, industrial	Central nervous system and mental effects

HAZARD	OCCUPATIONAL SOURCES	HEALTH EFFECTS
	measurement instruments, gold and silver refining	
Nickel	Nickel plating, steel manufacture, heating coils, hydrogenation processes	Lung and nasal cancer, skin effects
Tungsten	Steel manufacture, x-ray tubes	Lung and skin effects
Zinc oxide	White paint manufacture	Metal fume fever
Violence	Taxi driver, service station attendant, liquor or convenience store clerk, protective services personnel, jewelry clerks, fast food employees (working at night), security personnel	Trauma, homicide
Noise	Manufacturing, construction, grounds maintenance, work with heavy machinery	Hearing loss, stress
Pesticides	Agriculture, grounds maintenance	Respiratory and skin effects, neurological effects
Radiation	Mining, utilities, nuclear reactors, x-ray technicians, nuclear medicine	Lung and other cancers, radiation sickness
Stress	Jobs with low control, deadlines, shift work	Physical and mental effects
Sun exposure	Agriculture, forestry, logging, construction	Skin cancer
Trauma	Construction, logging, mining, trucking, agriculture, delivery services, transportation, utility work, manufacturing, sanitation, heavy lifting	Traumatic injury, musculoskeletal injury

▶ WORK FITNESS INVENTORY

Description: This inventory is intended for use in determining the individual employee's fitness for a specific job. The inventory incorporates elements of the biophysical, psychological, physical, social, behavioral, and health system dimensions of the Dimensions Model to assist health care providers in the occupational health setting to determine whether or not a given employee has the physical and mental capacity to perform certain tasks without endangering his or her health or the health and safety of others.

Appropriate populations: For use with individual employees.

Data sources and data collection strategies: Data may be obtained from interviews with employees and supervisors, specific tests of functional ability, laboratory test results, and review of the employee's job description. Additional data may be available from employee health records or from the records of other health care providers (with employee consent).

Use of information: Information derived from the inventory may be used to determine the appropriateness of initial hiring and placement decisions or an employee's fitness to return to work after an illness or injury. Information may also be used to help supervisors redesign an employee's position to prevent adverse health consequences. When information indicates a poor fit between the job and the employee, the nurse may also use this information to help the employee decide on career options that are more in keeping with his or her health status and capabilities.

▶ WORK FITNESS INVENTORY

BIOPHYSICAL DIMENSION CONSIDERATIONS	STATUS	
	Yes	No
Does the employee have the physical stamina required for the job?	☐	☐
Does the employee have any mobility limitations that would interfere with performance?	☐	☐
Does the employee have sufficient joint mobility to do the job?	☐	☐
Does the employee have any postural limitations that would interfere with performance?	☐	☐
Does the employee have the required strength for the job?	☐	☐
Does the employee have the level of coordination required?	☐	☐
Does the employee have problems with balance that would interfere with performance?	☐	☐
Does the employee have any cardiorespiratory limitations?	☐	☐
Is there a possibility for unconsciousness that would create a safety hazard?	☐	☐
Does the employee have the required level of visual and auditory acuity?	☐	☐
Does the employee have communication and speech capabilities required by the job?	☐	☐
Will the employee's age put him or her at increased risk of injury or illness?	☐	☐
Does the job involve shift work that will adversely affect biological rhythms?	☐	☐

PSYCHOLOGICAL DIMENSION CONSIDERATIONS		
Does the employee have the requisite level of cognitive function (eg, memory, critical thinking)?	☐	☐
Will the employee's mental or emotional state (eg, depression) interfere with performance?	☐	☐
Does the employee have the required motivational level?	☐	☐
Does the job involve high levels of stress?	☐	☐
Does the employee have effective stress management skills?	☐	☐
Does the employee have little control over his or her work?	☐	☐
Is there any possibility that the employee might endanger self or others?	☐	☐

PHYSICAL DIMENSION CONSIDERATIONS

Does the employee require assistive aids or appliances? Will work processes or setting need to be adapted to accommodate these aids (eg, space for a wheelchair)?	☐	☐
Are there risk factors in the work setting that would adversely affect the employee?	☐	☐
Does the job involve extreme weather exposures that would adversely affect the employee?	☐	☐
If the employee is pregnant or of childbearing age, are there reproductive risks present in the work setting or job activities?	☐	☐
Does the work setting pose problems for emergency evacuation of a disabled employee?	☐	☐

SOCIAL DIMENSION CONSIDERATIONS

Will the employee be working alone?	☐	☐
Will working alone have detrimental effects on the employee's physical or mental health?	☐	☐
Is the employee likely to be subjected to discrimination or sexual harassment?	☐	☐
Does the employee have the interpersonal skills required?	☐	☐
Does the job involve travel? Will travel adversely affect the employee's health?	☐	☐
Will travel or job schedule (eg, shift work) conflict with family responsibilities?	☐	☐

BEHAVIORAL DIMENSION CONSIDERATIONS

Does the employee have special dietary needs that cannot be met in the work setting?	☐	☐
Does the employee have a substance abuse problem that would interfere with performance?	☐	☐
Does the employee have a substance abuse problem that would pose a safety hazard to self or others?	☐	☐
Does the employee engage in behaviors (eg, smoking) that will interact negatively with other exposures in the work setting?	☐	☐
Does the job promote the necessary level of physical activity to maintain health?	☐	☐
Does the job involve strenuous physical activity beyond the employee's capability?	☐	☐
Does the employee have specific manual skills required for the job?	☐	☐

HEALTH SYSTEM DIMENSION CONSIDERATIONS

Are there treatment effects that will interfere with performance (eg, drowsiness due to medications)?	☐	☐
Will treatment plans interfere with performance (eg, nausea due to chemotherapy)?	☐	☐
What is the employee's prognosis? Will existing conditions improve or deteriorate?	☐	☐
Does the employee have any special health needs to be met in the work setting?	☐	☐

▶ OCCUPATIONAL HEALTH ASSESSMENT CONSIDERATIONS

- Factors inside and outside of the work setting may influence the health of employees, and the nurse should assess factors unrelated to the work setting that may contribute to health problems. The nurse should also consider the possibility of interactive effects between factors within and outside of the work setting.
- Employees may be reluctant to report health problems that they believe might jeopardize their employment. The nurse should be alert to signs and symptoms of health problems over and above those reported by employees.
- Employees may be particularly reluctant to admit to high-risk behaviors (eg, alcohol use) that may jeopardize their jobs. The nurse should ask about such behaviors in a matter-of-fact manner after informing employees of the need for the information. The nurse should also be alert to signs and symptoms of health problems caused by one's behavior or lifestyle. In addition, the nurse should investigate repeated or systematic work absences.
- Nurses may need to address ethical issues of confidentiality when employees' health problems place them or others at risk for injury.
- Employees may be resistant to routine health screenings, believing them unnecessary or disruptive to their work schedules. The nurse should educate the employee population regarding the need for and importance of routine screenings and engage in efforts to disrupt work schedules or personal time as little as possible.
- Employees may also resist use of safety equipment and procedures. Again, the nurse can be actively involved in educating employees regarding these practices. The nurse may need to work to get management to enforce safety procedures, and the nurse may need to monitor compliance with safety measures.
- In the course of assessing individual employees or employee populations, the nurse may identify hazardous conditions in the work setting. The nurse should be prepared to take these safety concerns to management or to regulatory agencies, if needed, to see that they are addressed.
- Employees' family problems may adversely affect their work performance, so the nurse should assess family interactions as well as other aspects of employees' health status. Although family members may not be officially sanctioned clients of the the nurse in the occupational health setting, the nurse may need to make referrals for services for family members to prevent their health problems from adversely affecting employee productivity.
- An occasional employee may make unfounded injury or illness claims related to the work setting. For this reason, the nurse must be particularly alert to discrepancies between an employee's reported symptoms and physical findings. The nurse should also be extremely diligent in accurately documenting all subjective and objective data, particularly with respect to injury events.

▶ HEALTH ASSESSMENT IN THE WORK SETTING

Description: This tool is intended to assist community health nurses working in occupational health settings to identify health problems present in employee populations. The tool also facilitates planning, implementation, and evaluation of nursing interventions for this population.

Appropriate populations: Groups of employees in business and industrial settings. May be applied to both manufacturing and service employment settings and with small or large groups of employees. Assessment of the health status of individual employees is better conducted using the *Health Assessment Guide—Adult Client* on page 93 of this handbook.

Data sources and data collection strategies: Data for assessing health needs in the occupational setting may be obtained from a variety of sources including company safety and injury records, employment compensation and insurance claims, employee health records, and interviews with employees and management personnel. Results of routine screening of employees also provide health status information. Health care providers in the community who provide services to employees may be another source of information. Additional information may be obtained through personal observation of working conditions, use of safety precautions, and so on. Because of the magnitude and complexity of the assessment data needed, the community health nurse may be one of several people collecting data. Community health nurses, however, are ideally suited to initiate and coordinate data collection as well as to guide the interpretation and use of the data obtained.

Use of information: Information on employee health status is used to derive community nursing diagnoses which direct the planning, implementation, and evaluation of health programs in the work setting. Information may also be used to identify larger community health concerns and to initiate efforts to address those concerns.

▶ HEALTH ASSESSMENT IN THE WORK SETTING

Biophysical Dimension

Age, sex, and racial/ethnic composition of the employee population: ____

Presence of handicapping conditions in the employee population: ____

Incidence and prevalence of disease *(communicable and chronic)*: ____

Prevalence of genetic predisposition to disease: ____

Extent of absenteeism: ____

Number and type of workers' compensation claims: ____

Immunization status *(diphtheria, tetanus, influenza, pneumonia)*: ____

Results of periodic screening tests: ____

Psychological Dimension

Organization of the work day *(shift work, breaks, overtime)*: ____

Aesthetic quality of environment: ____

Relationships among employees: ____

Relationships between employees and management: ____

Employee morale: ____

Supervisor leadership styles *(appropriateness)*: ____

Employee evaluation practices *(consistency, fairness)*: ____

Job satisfaction: ____

Extent of employee control of job: ____

Extent and sources of stress in the workplace: ____

Extent of work/home role conflict: ____

Availability of stress management programs: _____

Prevalence of emotional problems in the employee population: _____

Availability of employee assistance programs: _____

Physical Dimension
Typical commute *(distance, traffic)*: _____

Safety of parking areas: _____

Use of pesticides and other poisons in the work environment: _____

Pollutants in the work environment: _____

Fire or safety hazards: _____

Potential for toxic substance exposures: _____

Use of hazardous equipment: _____

Extent of exposure to extreme weather conditions: _____

Potential for falls: _____

Need for heavy lifting: _____

Ergonomics of workstations: _____

Animals/insects in the work environment: _____

Plant allergens or poisons in the work environment: _____

Adequacy of heating, lighting, cooling, ventilation: _____

Noise levels: _____

Sanitation of food preparation and storage areas: _____

Toilet facilities (*adequacy, state of repair*):_____

Availability of shower facilities for dealing with external toxic substance exposures: _____

Facilities and access for handicapped employees: _____

Potential for disaster: _____

Social Dimension

Economic stability of employing organization: _____

Salary levels *(adequacy, equity)*: _____

Health benefits available: _____

Community attitudes to employing organization: _____

Crime in neighborhood: _____

Potential for violence in the work setting: _____

Child care availability: _____

Family leave policies: _____

Intergroup conflicts/discrimination: _____

Cultural background of employees: _____

Languages spoken by employees: _____

Education level of employees and extent of health knowledge: _____

Coworker support for healthy behaviors: _____

Management support for healthy behaviors: _____

Implementation of safety legislation, regulations, policies: _____

Implementation of health-related policies: _____

Types of work performed and health effects: _____

Extent of sexual harassment: _____

Behavioral Dimension
CONSUMPTION PATTERNS
Nutritional quality of food services: _____

Employee nutrition levels: _____

Special nutrition needs: _____

Nutrition knowledge: _____

Extent of alcohol or drug use by employees: _____

Smoking *(extent, policies, cessation programs)*: _____

Medication use by employees: _____

LEISURE ACTIVITIES
Rest and activity patterns of employees: _____

Opportunity for physical activity: _____

OTHER
Adequacy of safety policies and procedures: _____

Use of appropriate safety equipment and procedures: _____

Health System Dimension
Health care services offered in work setting: _____

Availability of other health care services: _____

Use of health care services by employee population: _____

Funding of health care services *(adequacy, source)*: _____

Employee attitudes to health and health services: _____

Availability of health promotion programs: _____

Procedures to control and monitor toxic exposures: _____

Diagnosis

Biophysical Dimension

POPULATION HEALTH NEED/RISK	NEED–SERVICE MATCH/MISMATCH

Psychological Dimension

POPULATION HEALTH NEED/RISK	NEED–SERVICE MATCH/MISMATCH

Physical Dimension

POPULATION HEALTH NEED/RISK	NEED–SERVICE MATCH/MISMATCH

Social Dimension

POPULATION HEALTH NEED/RISK	NEED–SERVICE MATCH/MISMATCH

Behavioral Dimension

POPULATION HEALTH NEED/RISK	NEED–SERVICE MATCH/MISMATCH

Health System Dimension

POPULATION HEALTH NEED/RISK	NEED–SERVICE MATCH/MISMATCH

Planning

PLANNED INTERVENTIONS	OUTCOME OBJECTIVES

Implementation

INTERVENTION	RESPONSIBLE PARTY/ EXPECTED COMPLETION DATE	STATUS

Evaluation

EXPECTED OUTCOME	STATUS: MET/UNMET	SUPPORTING EVIDENCE

▶ DISASTER SETTINGS

Throughout history, people have been subjected to unexpected events that cause massive destruction, death, and injury. Almost any day of the week, the news media cover some kind of disaster somewhere in the world. Preparation for disasters and effective response when a disaster occurs can help minimize the long-term effect of these events.

Disasters are overwhelming events that exceed the ability of those affected to respond adequately. Disasters, natural or manmade, test the adaptive responses of communities or individuals beyond their capabilities and lead to at least a temporary disruption of function.

With their background in program planning and group dynamics, community health nurses are well suited to assist in developing disaster plans. Other roles they may perform include training rescue workers in triage techniques and basic first aid, educating those who will staff shelters about the needs of disaster victims, and educating the public regarding the community disaster plan and the need for personal preparation for a disaster. See *Nursing in the Community: Dimensions of Community Health Nursing* (Chapter 29) for and in-depth discussion of care in disaster settings.

▶ STAGES OF COMMUNITY DISASTER RESPONSE

Nondisaster Stage
- Identification of potential disaster risks
- Vulnerability analysis
- Resource inventory
- Prevention and mitigation
- Public and professional education

Predisaster Stage
- Warning
- Pre-impact mobilization
- Evacuation

Impact Stage
- Damage inventory
- Injury assessment

Emergency Stage
- Search and rescue
- First aid
- Emergency medical assistance
- Restoration of communication and transportation
- Public health surveillance
- Evacuation

Reconstruction Stage
- Restoration
- Reconstitution
- Mitigation

▶ AREAS FOR CLIENT EDUCATION RELATED TO DISASTER PREPAREDNESS

- Install and maintain smoke detectors in homes.
- Bolt bookcases and cabinets to walls in areas with earthquake potential.
- Determine avenues of escape from the home or other buildings.
- Install fire escape ladders as needed at upper windows.
- Keep stairways and doors free of obstacles to permit easy egress.
- Identify a place for family members to meet after escape from the home.
- Seek shelter in a reinforced area (eg, a doorway) during an earthquake and face away from windows. Stay indoors.
- Seek shelter from hurricanes or tornadoes in basements or inner rooms without windows.
- Seek high ground in the event of a flood.
- Drop to the ground and roll about to extinguish flaming clothing, or smother flames with a rug.
- Close doors and windows to prevent the spread of a fire, and place wadded fabric beneath doors to prevent smoke inhalation.
- Learn community disaster warning signals and their meaning.
- Know what actions should be taken when warning is given.
- Know where to seek additional information.
- Know the general plan for evacuating the community.
- Determine what valuables are to be taken if evacuation is required.
- Assign activities related to evacuation (eg, designate the person responsible for taking the baby or family pets).
- Know where proposed shelters will be located.
- Know where natural gas and water valves are located and how to turn them off. Attach a wrench close to valves.
- Keep a battery-operated radio and extra batteries available (replace batteries periodically).
- Designate a person living outside the area as a family contact if family members are separated during a disaster.
- Collect and store, in an accessible location, sufficient emergency supplies for 1 week, including:
    Nonperishable foods (including pet foods)
    Drinking water
    Warm clothing
    Bedding (blankets or sleeping bags)
    Tent or other type of shelter
    Source of light (flashlights or lanterns)
    Chlorine bleach for treating suspect water supplies to prevent infection
    First aid supplies and first aid manual
    Medications needed by family members
- Replace stored food, water, and medications periodically.

▶ COMMUNITY DISASTER PREPAREDNESS CHECKLIST

	YES	NO
Is there a community disaster plan? Is the plan being implemented?	☐	☐
Is there a person in charge of promoting, developing, and coordinating emergency preparation?	☐	☐
Does the disaster plan contain provisions for disaster warning to residents?	☐	☐
Are emergency preparedness activities coordinated among relevant community agencies?	☐	☐
Are all responding agencies and staff familiar with the community disaster plan?	☐	☐
Are community residents familiar with the disaster plan?	☐	☐
Are there operational plans for health response to a disaster?	☐	☐
Have mass casualty plans been developed by local health agencies?	☐	☐
Are surveillance measures in place for early detection and response to health emergencies?	☐	☐
Have steps been taken by environmental health services to prepare for disaster response?	☐	☐
Have facilities and safe areas been designated as shelter sites in the event of a disaster?	☐	☐
Have provisions been made for health care services in shelter sites?	☐	☐
Have health care personnel received disaster preparedness training?	☐	☐
Are resources available for rapid health response to disaster (eg, communications, financing, transport, supplies)?	☐	☐
Is there a system for updating information on supplies and personnel?	☐	☐
Has the disaster plan been tested?	☐	☐

▶ DISASTER ASSESSMENT AND PLANNING GUIDE

Description: This tool is intended to assist community health nurses and other community members to assess the level of disaster preparedness in the community and to plan for effective disaster response. The assessment component of the tool is based on the six dimensions of health in the Dimensions Model and reflects biophysical, psychological, physical, social, behavioral, and health system factors influencing disasters and community response to them. Community health nurses and others assessing community disaster preparedness may want to begin the assessment with the *Community Disaster Preparedness Checklist* (see page 192 of this handbook) to identify areas in which more in-depth assessment is required and then use this tool to direct that in-depth assessment.

Appropriate populations: The tool may be used to assess and plan for disaster preparedness at the community level. It may also be used to develop disaster plans for specific health care agencies and institutions or other groups within the community (eg, schools).

Data sources and data collection strategies: Sources of data for community disaster assessment and planning may include community historical records, official government documents, existing disaster plans of community agencies and organizations, and interviews with key individuals within the community. Additional sources of data may include local businesses and industries, schools, health departments, civil defense/disaster agencies, and the local Chapter of the American Red Cross. Information on community resources may also be available from social and civic organizations and clubs. Area maps and personal observation by the community health nurse and others may also provide important information. Because disaster planning should be a community-wide endeavor, community health nurses will be only one group involved in obtaining assessment data and developing a community disaster plan. Community health nurses, however, may create the impetus for disaster planning and/or coordinate data collection and interpretation and disaster response planning.

Use of information: Data obtained using the tool will be used to identify community disaster potential and to plan means of preventing disasters from occurring or mitigating their adverse effects on the community. Assessment data should be used to develop a general plan of community disaster response that would fit many types of disaster events. Assessment data may also serve as an impetus for educating the general public regarding disaster preparedness.

▶ DISASTER ASSESSMENT AND PLANNING GUIDE

Assessment

Biophysical Dimension

What is the age composition of the population(s) most likely to be affected by a disaster? _____

Are there special health needs present in the age group(s) identified? _____

What is the ethnic/racial composition of the population(s) most likely to be affected by a disaster? What effects, if any, will ethnicity have on response to a disaster? _____

What is the extent of injury anticipated as a result of a disaster? What types of injuries are most likely to occur? _____

What chronic health problems are prevalent among the population(s) most likely to be affected by a disaster? _____

What communicable disease problems are anticipated as a result of a disaster? _____

What currently existing communicable diseases prevalent in the community might complicate disaster response and recovery (eg, TB, HIV infection)? _____

What is the typical rate of pregnancy in the population(s) most likely to be affected by a disaster? _____

Psychological Dimension

What is the attitude of members of the community to disaster preparedness? _____

How has the community responded to disasters in the past, if any? _____

What is the response of community members to disaster warnings? What factors are influencing their response? _____

What is the extent of the community's ability to cope with the effects of a disaster? _____

What is the prevalence of mental illness in the population(s) most likely to be affected by a disaster? _____

What effect is the extent of mental illness likely to have on community disaster response? _____

Physical Dimension

What physical features of the community create the potential for disaster? Is there potential for:
Flooding: _____

Forest or brushfires: _____

Earthquake: _____

Explosion or volcanic eruption: _____

Severe weather conditions: _____

What structures are most/least likely to be damaged in a disaster? _____

To what extent are vital community structures likely to withstand a disaster? _____

What community structures could be used as emergency shelters? _____

What effect are local weather conditions likely to have on community response to a disaster? _____

Are there elements of the physical environment that might hinder disaster response (eg, blockage of roads)? _____

Is it likely that a disaster event will threaten community water supplies? _____

Are animals likely to be involved in a disaster? If so, what effect will this have on human health? _____

Social Dimension

Do relationships in the community have the potential to create a disaster (eg, war, civil strife)? _____

How cohesive is the community? Are community members able to work together for disaster planning? _____

Is there potential for conflict between populations most likely to be affected by a disaster? _____

What provisions, if any, have been made for reuniting families separated by a disaster? _____

What social support systems will be available to victims if a disaster occurs? _____

To what extent do community agencies collaborate in disaster planning? _____

What is the extent of knowledge among community residents regarding plans for disaster response? _____

What plans have been made for communicating disaster warnings to residents? _____

Is there a need for special measures to communicate warnings to some groups in the community? If so, what factors contribute to these special needs? _____

Are there language barriers to communicating disaster warnings? If so, have plans been made to circumvent these barriers? _____

What are the anticipated effects of a disaster on normal channels of communication in the community? _____

What community group/agency is responsible for coordinating disaster planning? _____

How widespread is community participation in disaster planning? _____

Who is responsible for activating the community disaster plan? How will this person be notified of a disaster? _____

Do community leaders responsible for disaster response activities have high levels of credibility among residents? _____

Do community industries pose disaster hazards? If so, what types of hazards are involved? _____

To what extent do local industries adhere to safety standards? How is adherence monitored? _____

What occupational groups present in the community could assist with disaster response? How will these groups be notified of the need for their assistance? _____

How adequate is the number of rescue personnel available to meet community disaster needs? _____

How adequately have rescue personnel been trained in rescue operations? Is their training updated periodically? _____

What is the extent of the community's economic capacity for recovery after a disaster? _____

What economic assistance is anticipated following a disaster? How might it be obtained? _____

What are the anticipated effects of different types of disasters on the local economy? _____

Is there potential for transportation-related disaster? _____

What is the anticipated effect of a disaster on local transportation? _____

What is the anticipated effect of a disaster on essential community services? _____

What equipment is available for disaster response? Is it kept in good working order? _____

Have anticipated supplies for effective disaster response been stored at accessible locations throughout the community? Are supplies replaced as needed? _____

Behavioral Dimension

Do consumption patterns (eg, smoking, alcohol use) create the potential for disaster? _____

What is the extent of substance use and abuse in the community? What effect will this have on community disaster response? _____

Have plans been made to provide food and water for anticipated disaster victims and rescuers? _____

How will food and water supplies be dispensed? _____

Are there special dietary needs among the population(s) likely to be affected by a disaster? What provisions have been made to meet those needs? _____

What community leisure pursuits pose potential disaster hazards? _____

Do community members engage in recreational safety measures designed to prevent disasters? _____

What leisure pursuits by community members could enhance disaster response capabilities? _____

Health System Dimension

How well prepared are health service agencies to respond to a disaster? ___

What facilities are available to care for disaster victims? _____

What is the extent of basic first aid and other health-related knowledge in the community? _____

What health care personnel are available to meet health needs in a disaster (*consider both emergency and routine service needs*)? How will they be mobilized to respond? _____

What is the anticipated effect of a disaster on health care services? What steps have been taken to minimize disruption of services? _____

What health care needs are anticipated as a result of a disaster? What plans have been made to meet those needs? _____

What plans have been made to support triage activities? _____

What plans have been made for creating medical treatment areas? for transporting victims to these areas? _____

What medications are likely to be needed by victims of a disaster? Have supplies of essential medications been stored in accessible locations? _____

What medical and first aid supplies will be needed for disaster response? for health care in shelters? Have these supplies been obtained and stored in accessible locations? _____

How will medications and supplies be transported to areas of need? How will they be dispensed? _____

Have plans been made for the identification of the dead? for notifying family members? for disposing of bodies? _____

What mental health services will be available immediately following a disaster and during the recovery period? _____

Diagnosis and Planning
Community Disaster Potential

TYPE OF POTENTIAL DISASTER	CONTRIBUTING FACTORS

Vulnerable Populations

POPULATION	SOURCE OF VULNERABILITY

Disaster Prevention/Mitigation Activities

DISASTER PREVENTION ACTIVITIES	DISASTER MITIGATION ACTIVITIES

Anticipated Disaster-related Health Problems and Planned Interventions

ANTICIPATED PROBLEM	PLANNED INTERVENTION

Disaster Plan Elements

Mechanisms for warning residents: _____
_____

Mechanisms for initiating disaster plan implementation: _____

Plans for communication: _____
_____

Procedures for traffic control and transportation of equipment, supplies, and personnel to the disaster site: _____
_____

Procedures for evacuating residents: _____
_____
_____

Plans for rescue operations: _____

Plans for damage inventory: _____

Plans for mobilizing health providers: _____

Plans for injury assessment: _____

Plans for meeting immediate care needs of disaster victims: _____

Plans for providing shelter: _____

Plans for shelter governance: _____

Plans for providing supportive care: _____

Plans for public health surveillance: _____

Mechanisms to assist victims during the recovery period: _____

Mechanisms for evaluating the adequacy of the disaster plan: _____

SECTION VI

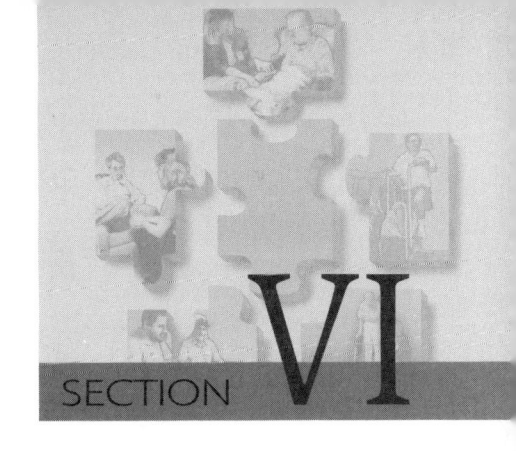

COMMON COMMUNITY HEALTH PROBLEMS

▶ **COMMUNICABLE DISEASES**

Infectious diseases are a leading cause of death throughout the world. New diseases are emerging, and others thought to be controlled are resurfacing. Several factors contribute to the emergence of disease. Societal changes, such as war, population growth, and urban deterioration, have increased people's susceptibility. Environmental changes, such as deforestation, expose previously hidden animal reservoirs of disease. Human behaviors, such as global travel, sexual promiscuity, and drug use, also lead to exposure to infectious agents. Moreover, within the health care system the use and abuse of antimicrobial agents is a factor, as is reduced funding for communicable disease control programs.

Community health nurses work to prevent, identify, and control communicable diseases. See *Nursing in the Community: Dimensions of Community Health Nursing* (Chapter 30) for a full discussion of the role of community health nurses in communicable disease control.

▶ PORTALS OF ENTRY AND EXIT FOR EACH MODE OF DISEASE TRANSMISSION

MODE OF TRANSMISSION	PORTAL OF ENTRY	PORTAL OF EXIT
Airborne	Respiratory system	Respiratory system
Fecal–oral	Mouth	Feces
Direct contact	Skin, mucous membrane	Skin, mucous membrane
Sexual contact	Skin, mouth, urethra, vagina, rectum	Skin lesions, vaginal or urethral secretions
Direct inoculation	Across placenta, bloodstream	Blood
Animal or insect bite	Wound in skin	Blood, saliva
Other means of transmission	Wound in skin, intact skin	Animal feces, soil

▶ INFORMATION ON SELECTED COMMUNICABLE DISEASES

Chlamydia

Agent: Chlamydia trachomatis
Reservoir: Humans
Incubation: Probably 7–14 days
Communicability: Unknown, relapse possible
Modes of transmission: Sexual contact
Immunization: None
Prophylaxis: Antibiotics following sexual exposure or for infants born to infected mothers
Treatment: Tetracycline, doxycycline, erythromycin, or azithromycin
Contact notification: Sexual contacts
Symptoms: Frequently asymptomatic; *males* may have urethritis with burning on urination, urethral itching, penile discharge; *females* may have purulent vaginal discharge
Prevention: Monogamy, condom use

Coccidioidomycosis

Agent: Coccidioides immitis (fungus)
Reservoir: Soil
Incubation: 1–4 weeks
Communicability: No person-to-person transmission

Modes of transmission: Inhalation of contaminated dust
Immunization: None
Prophylaxis: None
Treatment: Usually self-limiting; amphotericin B for severe infection, fluconazole for meningeal infection, ketoconazole or itraconazole for chronic infection
Contact notification: None
Symptoms: Asymptomatic or fever, cough, chills
Prevention: Dust control measures

Diphtheria (Pharyngotonsillar, Laryngeal)

Agent: Corynebacterium diphtheriae
Reservoir: Humans
Incubation: 2–5 days
Communicability: Usually 2 weeks or less, reduced by antibiotic therapy
Modes of transmission: Airborne, raw milk, contact with articles soiled with discharge from lesions (rare)
Immunization: Routine use of DTP vaccine (Td for persons over age 7)
Prophylaxis: Penicillin or erythromycin and booster dose of diphtheria toxoid or full immunization series
Treatment: Diphtheria antitoxin and penicillin or erythromycin
Contact notification: None
Symptoms: Sore throat with patchy, grayish membrane over pharynx, tonsils, uvula, and soft palate; cervical lymphadenopathy
Prevention: Immunization of susceptible individuals

Gonorrhea

Agent: Neisseria gonorrhoeae
Reservoir: Humans
Incubation: Usually 2–7 days
Communicability: Until treated
Modes of transmission: Sexual contact
Immunization: None
Prophylaxis: Antibiotics after exposure
Treatment: Ceftriaxone and doxycycline
Contact notification: Sexual contacts
Symptoms: Vary with site of infection; usually associated with penile discharge and burning on urination in urethritis in males and with anal discharge, tenesmus, and pruritis in rectal infection; may be associated with vaginal discharge and foul odor in females; sore throat in oral infection
Prevention: Monogamy, use of condoms

Hantavirus (Pulmonary)

Agent: Hantavirus (multiple strains)
Reservoir: Rodents
Incubation: 2 weeks
Communicability: No person-to-person transmission
Modes of transmission: Inhalation of dust contaminated with urine, feces, saliva of infected rodents
Immunization: None
Prophylaxis: None
Treatment: Symptomatic
Contact notification: None
Symptoms: Fever, myalgias, chills, nonproductive cough, headache, nausea, vomiting, diarrhea, malaise; may progress to fulminant adult respiratory distress syndrome (ARDS) in severe cases
Prevention: Rodent control, proper cleaning and disposal of rodent excreta

Hepatitis A

Agent: Hepatitis A virus (HAV)
Reservoir: Humans, nonhuman primates
Incubation: Average 28–30 days
Communicability: Latter half of incubation period to a few days after onset of jaundice
Modes of transmission: Fecal–oral, sexual contact (homosexual males), contaminated food or water, direct inoculation (rare)
Immunization: Hepatitis A vaccine
Prophylaxis: Immunoglobulin (Ig)
Treatment: Symptomatic
Contact notification: Household and sexual contacts, day-care center classroom contacts
Symptoms: Abrupt onset of fever, malaise, anorexia, nausea and vomiting, abdominal discomfort followed by jaundice; adults more likely to be symptomatic than children
Prevention: Sanitation, personal hygiene (handwashing), adequate cooking of contaminated foods

Hepatitis B

Agent: Hepatitis B virus (HBV)
Reservoir: Humans
Incubation: Average 60–90 days
Communicability: Several weeks before and after symptom onset; may be lifelong carrier

Modes of transmission: Sexual contact, direct inoculation, transplacental
Immunization: Hepatitis B vaccine
Prophylaxis: Hepatitis B immunoglobulin and/or immunization
Treatment: Symptomatic, alfa-interferon for chronic infection
Contact notification: Household or sexual contacts, intravenous drug partners
Symptoms: Insidious onset of anorexia, abdominal discomfort, nausea and vomiting, followed by jaundice
Prevention: Immunization of infants and persons in high-risk groups; monogamy, condom use, blood donor screening, drug abuse treatment; avoid needle sharing; blood and body fluid precautions

Hepatitis C

Agent: Hepatitis C virus (HCV)
Reservoir: Humans
Incubation: Average 6–9 weeks
Communicability: 1 or more weeks prior to onset through acute clinical phase
Modes of transmission: Direct inoculation, sexual contact
Immunization: None
Prophylaxis: None
Treatment: Symptomatic, alpha-interferon for chronic infection
Contact notification: Intravenous drug partners
Symptoms: Insidious onset of anorexia, vague abdominal discomfort, nausea and vomiting, jaundice
Prevention: Same as for hepatitis B

Hepatitis D (Delta)

Agent: Hepatitis D virus (HDV)
Reservoir: Humans
Incubation: 2–8 weeks
Communicability: Prior to onset through acute clinical phase
Modes of transmission: Direct inoculation, sexual contact
Immunization: None
Prophylaxis: None
Treatment: Symptomatic
Contact notification: None
Symptoms: Abrupt onset of symptoms similar to HBV; always associated with coexistent HBV infection
Prevention: Same as for hepatitis B

Hepatitis E

Agent: Hepatitis E virus (HEV)
Reservoir: Humans
Incubation: 26–42 days
Communicability: Unknown
Modes of transmission: Fecal–oral, contaminated water
Immunization: None
Prophylaxis: None
Treatment: Symptomatic
Contact notification: None
Symptoms: Similar to HAV
Prevention: Sanitation, hygiene

HIV Infection

Agent: Human immunodeficiency virus (HIV)
Reservoir: Humans
Incubation: 2 months to 10 years
Communicability: Unknown; presumed lifelong
Modes of transmission: Sexual contact, direct inoculation, transplacental inoculation, breastfeeding
Immunization: None
Prophylaxis: Antiviral agents
Treatment: Antiviral agents
Contact notification: Sexual partners, intravenous drug partners, clients of infected health care professionals, recipients of blood or tissue from infected donors
Symptoms: Fatigue, malaise, recurrent and sustained opportunistic infections
Prevention: Monogamy, condom use, drug treatment; avoid needle sharing; screen blood and organ donors

HSV Infection

Agent: Herpes simplex virus (HSV) type 2
Reservoir: Humans
Incubation: 2–12 days
Communicability: 7–12 days, initial lesion; 4–7 days, recurrent lesions
Modes of transmission: Sexual contact
Immunization: None
Prophylaxis: None
Treatment: Symptomatic; acyclovir
Contact notification: Pregnant women

Symptoms: Painful genital lesions
Prevention: Monogamy, condom use

Influenza

Agent: Influenza viruses A, B, C
Reservoir: Humans (animals for new subtypes)
Incubation: 1–3 days
Communicability: 3–7 days after onset of symptoms
Modes of transmission: Airborne
Immunization: Annual use of influenza vaccine for high-risk individuals
Prophylaxis: Amantidine or rimantidine in high-risk persons (type A only)
Treatment: Symptomatic, amantidine or rimantidine within 48 hours of onset
Contact notification: None
Symptoms: Fever, headache, myalgia, prostration, coryza, sore throat, cough, nausea, vomiting, diarrhea
Prevention: Immunization of persons at risk; general health promotion

Lyme Disease

Agent: Borrelia burgdorferi
Reservoir: Wild rodents, deer ticks
Incubation: 3–32 days
Communicability: No person-to-person transmission
Modes of transmission: Bite of infected tick
Immunization: None
Prophylaxis: None
Treatment: Doxycycline, amoxicillin
Contact notification: Source case finding if outside endemic areas
Symptoms: Distinctive skin lesion, followed by malaise, fatigue, fever, headache, stiff neck, myalgias, migratory arthralgia, lymphadenopathy
Prevention: Use insect repellant, wear long-sleeved, light-colored clothes, check for ticks regularly; tick control measures

Measles

Agent: Measles virus
Reservoir: Humans
Incubation: Average 10 days
Communicability: Beginning of prodrome to 4 days after onset of rash
Modes of transmission: Airborne
Immunization: Routine use of measles, mumps, rubella (MMR) vaccine
Prophylaxis: MMR within 72 hours of exposure; measles immunoglobulin for children under 1 year within 6 days of exposure

Treatment: Symptomatic
Contact notification: None
Symptoms: Prodrome of fever, conjunctivitis, cough, coryza, and Koplik's spots, followed by rash on face and spreading downward
Prevention: Routine immunization of all susceptible individuals

Mumps

Agent: Mumps virus
Reservoir: Humans
Incubation: Usually 18 days
Communicability: 6–7 days before swelling to 9 days after
Modes of transmission: Airborne
Immunization: Routine use of measles, mumps, rubella (MMR) vaccine
Prophylaxis: None
Treatment: Symptomatic
Contact notification: None
Symptoms: Pain and swelling in parotid area accompanied by difficulty swallowing; redness and swelling around Stensen's duct
Prevention: Immunization of susceptible individuals

Pertussis

Agent: Bordetella pertussis
Reservoir: Humans
Incubation: 7–10 days
Communicability: Early catarrhal stage to 3 weeks after cough begins
Modes of transmission: Airborne
Immunization: Routine use of diphtheria/tetanus/pertussis (DTP) vaccine
Prophylaxis: DTP booster and erythromycin
Treatment: Erythromycin may reduce communicability
Contact notification: Nonimmune children
Symptoms: Initial catarrhal stage followed by paroxysmal whooping cough
Prevention: Immunization of susceptible individuals

Poliomyelitis

Agent: Poliovirus types 1, 2, 3
Reservoir: Humans
Incubation: 7–14 days
Communicability: Unknown, possible 36–72 hours after exposure to 10 days after symptoms occur
Modes of transmission: Airborne, contaminated milk and food

Immunization: Routine use of trivalent inactivated polio vaccine (IPV) and oral polio vaccine (OPV)
Prophylaxis: None
Treatment: Symptomatic
Contact notification: Close contacts
Symptoms: Fever, headache, gastrointestinal disturbance, stiffness of neck and back with or without paralysis
Prevention: Immunization of susceptible children; sanitation

Rubella

Agent: Rubella virus
Reservoir: Humans
Incubation: 16–18 days
Communicability: 1 week before to 4 days after onset of rash
Modes of transmission: Airborne, transplacental inoculation
Immunization: Routine use of measles, mumps, rubella (MMR) vaccine
Prophylaxis: Immunoglobulin (Ig) for pregnant women (value ?)
Treatment: Symptomatic
Contact notification: Pregnant women
Symptoms: Prodrome of mild fever, headache, and malaise, followed by discrete maculopapular rash, occipital node enlargement
Prevention: Immunization of susceptible individuals, especially women of childbearing age

Syphilis

Agent: Treponema pallidum
Reservoir: Humans
Incubation: 10–90 days (usually 3 weeks)
Communicability: In stages with lesions
Modes of transmission: Sexual contact, direct inoculation, transplacental inoculation
Immunization: None
Prophylaxis: Antibiotics after exposure
Treatment: Penicillin
Contact notification: Sexual contacts to primary, secondary, and early latent syphilis; persons sharing needles
Symptoms: Vary with stage of disease
- *Primary:* Painless chancre or lesion at site of infection (usually genitalia, lips, etc.); may be accompanied by localized lymphadenopathy in the area of the lesion
- *Secondary:* Coppery, macular rash (may be found in all areas but particu-

larly on palms and soles); may be accompanied by malaise and generalized lymphadenopathy
- *Latent:* Asymptomatic
- *Late:* Depends on organ system affected
- *Congenital:* Hutchinson's teeth and raspberry molars, saddle nose, snuffles, rash if in secondary stage

Prevention: Monogamy, condom use, drug abuse treatment; avoid needle sharing; screening of blood donors

Tetanus

Agent: Clostridium tetani
Reservoir: Humans and animals, soil
Incubation: 3–21 days
Communicability: Not directly communicable
Modes of transmission: Introduction via wound in skin or unhealed umbilicus
Immunization: Routine use of diphtheria/tetanus/pertussis (DTP) vaccine
Prophylaxis: Tetanus/diphtheria (Td) booster for immunized persons; tetanus immunoglobulin (TIg) or tetanus antitoxin and Td for unimmunized individuals
Treatment: TIg or antitoxin and penicillin
Contact notification: None
Symptoms: Painful muscular contractions with progressive rigidity, especially in muscles of neck and shoulders
Prevention: Immunization of susceptible individuals, prevent injury, cleanse injuries thoroughly, control animal feces; asepsis during deliveries

Tuberculosis

Agent: Mycobacterium tuberculosis
Reservoir: Humans, cattle, other animals
Incubation: 4–12 weeks
Communicability: During periods of respiratory expulsion of bacteria
Modes of transmission: Airborne, contaminated milk
Immunization: Bacille Calmette–Guerin (BCG) for selected individuals
Prophylaxis: Isoniazid
Treatment: Antituberculin agents (multidrug regimen)
Contact notification: Close contacts
Symptoms: Cough, hemoptysis, unexplained weight loss, night sweats
Prevention: Improve social conditions, promote general health

▶ COMMUNICABLE DISEASE RISK FACTOR INVENTORY

Description: This inventory is intended to assist the community health nurse to identify clients at risk for communicable diseases. Risk factors in each of the six dimensions of health are addressed.

Appropriate populations: May be used with individual clients or population groups to identify risk factors amenable to modification. Appropriate to all age groups and cultural groups.

Data sources and data collection strategies: For individual clients, most of the information addressed in the inventory will be obtained from interviews with the client or significant others. Some information may also be available in existing health records (eg, history of treatment for sexually transmitted disease). Information related to population groups will come from a variety of sources including local health department statistics, records of local health care providers, school records, and data on absenteeism from local industries and businesses. Additional information may be obtained in interviews with or surveys of community residents or major informants such as health care providers, community officials, and so on.

Use of information: Risk factors identified in the use of the inventory provide a starting point for client education and efforts to modify risk factors to prevent the occurrence of communicable diseases or to limit their effects on individuals or population groups. Based on his or her knowledge of the contribution of specific types of risk factors for certain communicable diseases, the community health nurse explores with the client the risk of communicable disease and ways to modify risk factors to prevent disease or mitigate its effects. For example, if the client has multiple sexual partners and uses injecting drugs, the community health nurse would determine that this individual is at high risk for HIV infection, hepatitis B, C, and D, and sexually transmitted diseases. The nurse would then educate the client regarding the increased risk of these diseases and suggest ways of eliminating or modifying risk factors.

▶ COMMUNICABLE DISEASE RISK FACTOR INVENTORY

(Note: The "client" may be an individual or a group of people) **YES   NO**

BIOPHYSICAL DIMENSION

- Is the client (population) in an age group at particular risk for:
  - Measles? ☐ ☐
  - Mumps? ☐ ☐
  - Rubella? ☐ ☐
  - Diphtheria? ☐ ☐
  - Pertussis? ☐ ☐
  - Tetanus? ☐ ☐
  - Poliomyelitis? ☐ ☐
  - HiB disease? ☐ ☐
  - Hepatitis A? ☐ ☐
  - Hepatitis B? ☐ ☐
  - HIV infection? ☐ ☐
  - Sexually transmitted diseases? ☐ ☐
  - Tuberculosis? ☐ ☐
  - Influenza? ☐ ☐
  - Varicella? ☐ ☐
- Does the client have an existing chronic disease? ☐ ☐
- Is the client receiving immunosuppressive therapy? ☐ ☐
- Does the client have HIV infection? ☐ ☐
- Is the client overly fatigued? ☐ ☐
- Is the client pregnant? ☐ ☐
- Does the client have a history of sexually transmitted diseases? ☐ ☐
- Has the client received blood or blood products? ☐ ☐

PSYCHOLOGICAL DIMENSION

- Is the client under stress? ☐ ☐
- Is the client depressed? ☐ ☐
- Does the client have a poor self-image that would lead to high-risk behaviors? ☐ ☐

PHYSICAL DIMENSION

- Does the client live in crowded conditions? ☐ ☐
- Is the client at risk for insect or animal bites? ☐ ☐
- Do physical environmental conditions contribute to the presence of disease vectors? ☐ ☐
- Is the client exposed to contaminated food or water? ☐ ☐
- Is the client exposed to poor sanitary conditions? ☐ ☐

SOCIAL DIMENSION | YES | NO

- Is the client homeless? ☐ ☐
- Does the client live in a shelter or other institutional setting? ☐ ☐
- Is the client subjected to peer pressure for high-risk behaviors? ☐ ☐
- Do social mores support high-risk behaviors? ☐ ☐
- Are family members or friends ill? ☐ ☐
- Does the client's occupation increase the risk of disease? ☐ ☐
- If in a high-risk occupation, does the client use universal precautions? ☐ ☐
- Is the client involved in child care (*as recipient or provider*)? ☐ ☐
- Do cultural beliefs and behaviors increase the client's risk of disease? ☐ ☐
- Does the client live in an area where communicable disease is endemic? ☐ ☐
- Does the client travel to areas where communicable disease is endemic? ☐ ☐

BEHAVIORAL DIMENSION

- Is the client malnourished? ☐ ☐
- Does the client engage in substance abuse? ☐ ☐
- Does the client use injectable drugs? ☐ ☐
- Does the client share drug paraphernalia? ☐ ☐
- Does the client frequent "shooting galleries"? ☐ ☐
- Is the client sexually active? ☐ ☐
- Does the client have multiple sexual partners? ☐ ☐
- Does the client use safe sexual practices? ☐ ☐
- Does the client engage in regular condom use with sexual activity? ☐ ☐
- Does the client douche? ☐ ☐
- Does the client use oral contraceptives? ☐ ☐
- Does the client engage in prostitution for drugs or money? ☐ ☐
- Does the client have sexual intercourse with members of high-risk groups? ☐ ☐
- Does the client use good personal hygiene practices (eg, handwashing)? ☐ ☐
- Does the client wash fruits and vegetables thoroughly before eating them? ☐ ☐
- Does the client cook foods sufficiently to kill any microorganisms? ☐ ☐
- Does the client purify contaminated water before drinking or cooking? ☐ ☐

HEALTH SYSTEM DIMENSION	YES	NO
• Is the client adequately immunized against:		
Measles?	☐	☐
Mumps?	☐	☐
Rubella?	☐	☐
Diphtheria?	☐	☐
Pertussis?	☐	☐
Tetanus?	☐	☐
HiB disease?	☐	☐
Hepatitis A?	☐	☐
Hepatitis B?	☐	☐
Varicella?	☐	☐
Influenza?	☐	☐
Tuberculosis?	☐	☐
• Can the client afford immunization services?	☐	☐
• Does the client's insurance cover immunization services?	☐	☐

▶ COMMUNICABLE DISEASE RISK FACTOR MODIFICATION STRATEGIES

RISK FACTOR	STRATEGIES FOR MODIFICATION
Biophysical Dimension	
Presence of existing disease	Treat or control existing disease (eg, treat syphilis to decrease risk of HIV infection)
Immunosuppressive therapy	Provide prophylactic antibiotics, isolation procedures
Fatigue	Encourage rest
Pregnancy	Avoid known exposure to communicable diseases
Psychological Dimension	
Stress	Reduce stress levels if possible, teach coping skills
Poor self-image	Enhance self-image
Depression	Refer for treatment of depression
Physical Dimension	
Crowded living conditions	Refer for housing assistance, promote adequate ventilation, use of ultraviolet light
Insect/animal bite	Encourage protective clothing, insect repellent, avoid wild animals if possible, vector control strategies
Contaminated food or water	Wash foods before eating, cook sufficiently, boil water
Poor sanitary conditions	Refer for assistance with improving sanitation
Social Dimension	
Homelessness	Refer for shelter, long-term housing
Shelter/institutional living	Encourage use of ultraviolet light, promote adequate ventilation, use of universal precautions
Peer pressure for risk behavior	Teach good coping skills, assertiveness
Social mores	Change societal attitudes to unhealthful behaviors
Occupational risk	Promote universal precautions
Child care	Enforce exclusion of sick children, promote good hygiene
Travel	Provide needed immunizations, encourage care in eating and drinking

RISK FACTOR	STRATEGIES FOR MODIFICATION
Behavioral Dimension	
Malnutrition	Improve nutritional status, educate on nutritional needs, assist with food budget, if needed
Substance abuse	Refer for treatment if desired, educate regarding needle-sharing
Unsafe sexual activity	Encourage safer sexual practices, use of barrier contraceptives, limiting number of sexual partners, partner selectivity
Douching	Encourage to discontinue douching
Poor hygiene	Encourage handwashing
Health System Dimension	
Lack of immunization	Refer for or provide immunizations, refer for financial assistance as needed

▶ CHRONIC PHYSICAL HEALTH PROBLEMS

Because of the effectiveness of control measures developed for many previously fatal communicable diseases, chronic health problems have largely replaced communicable diseases as the leading causes of death and disability in the United States. Chronic health problems are those that are present for extended periods and that are characterized by one or more distinctive features. These features may include nonreversible pathological changes, a need for lifestyle adjustment, or a prolonged period of supervision and care by health professionals. Chronic conditions are also frequently characterized by disability—an inability to perform one or more functions of everyday life satisfactorily.

Community health nurses are actively involved in several aspects of efforts to control the effects of chronic health problems for both individuals and their families and for the population-at-large. Roles played by community health nurses in chronic disease control include caregiver, educator, counselor, advocate, case manager, researcher, and role model. They identify factors that place individuals or communities at risk for problems related to chronic conditions and take action to modify those factors. Additionally, they might identify persons with existing chronic conditions and assist them to deal with problems related to their disease. See *Nursing in the Community: Dimensions of Community Health Nursing* (Chapter 31) for an in-depth presentation of chronic physical health problems.

▶ CHRONIC DISEASE RISK FACTOR INVENTORY

Description: This inventory is intended to assist the community health nurse to identify clients at risk for common chronic conditions. Risk factors in each of the six dimensions of health are addressed.

Appropriate populations: May be used with individual clients or population groups to identify risk factors amenable to modification. Appropriate to all age groups and cultural groups.

Data sources and data collection strategies: For individual clients, most of the information addressed in the inventory will be obtained from interviews with the client or significant others. Some information may also be available in existing health records. Information related to population groups will come from a variety of sources including local health department statistics, records of local health care providers, school records, and data on absenteeism from local industries and businesses. Additional information may be obtained in interviews with or surveys of community residents or major informants such as health care providers, community officials, and so on.

Use of information: Risk factors identified in the use of the inventory provide a starting point for client education and efforts to modify risk factors to prevent the occurrence of chronic conditions or to limit their effects on individuals or population groups. Based on his or her knowledge of the contribution of specific types of risk factors for certain chronic conditions, the community health nurse explores with the client the risk of disease and ways to modify risk factors to prevent disease or mitigate its effects. For example, if the client has a family history of lung cancer and smokes, the community health nurse would determine that this individual is at high risk for lung cancer and other chronic conditions such as heart disease. The nurse would then educate the client regarding the increased risk of these diseases and suggest ways of eliminating or modifying risk factors.

▶ CHRONIC DISEASE RISK FACTOR INVENTORY

(Note: The "client" may be an individual or a group of people) **YES   NO**

BIOPHYSICAL DIMENSION

- Is the client (population) in an age group at particular risk for chronic health problems? ☐ ☐
- Does the client have a family history of hereditary chronic health problems? ☐ ☐
- Does the client have an existing condition that increases the risk of other chronic problems? ☐ ☐
- Does the client have physical problems that increase the risk of accidental injury? ☐ ☐
- Is the client overweight? ☐ ☐
- Does the client have hypertension? ☐ ☐
- Does the client have asthma or RAD? ☐ ☐

PSYCHOLOGICAL DIMENSION

- Is the client under stress? ☐ ☐

PHYSICAL DIMENSION

- Is the client exposed to environmental pollutants? ☐ ☐
- Do environmental conditions increase the risk of accidental injury? ☐ ☐
- Is the client exposed to high noise levels? ☐ ☐
- Is the client exposed to temperature extremes? ☐ ☐
- Is the client exposed to high levels of ionizing radiation? ☐ ☐

SOCIAL DIMENSION   YES   NO

- Do societal norms support behaviors that increase the risk of chronic health problems? ☐ ☐
- Do the client's peers support behaviors that increase the risk of chronic problems? ☐ ☐
- Do cultural beliefs and behaviors increase the risk of chronic health problems? ☐ ☐
- Does legislation affect the risk of chronic health problems? ☐ ☐
- Does the client's occupation increase the risk of disease? ☐ ☐
- If in a high-risk occupation, does the client engage in preventive measures at work? ☐ ☐

BEHAVIORAL DIMENSION

- Does the client's diet increase the risk of chronic health problems? ☐ ☐
- Does the client smoke? ☐ ☐
- Does the client use drugs or alcohol that increase the risk of chronic health problems? ☐ ☐
- Does the client have a sedentary lifestyle? ☐ ☐
- Do self-care practices (eg, BSE or TSE) decrease the risk of death from chronic health problems? ☐ ☐
- Do sexual practices increase the risk of chronic health problems (eg, multiple sexual partners increases risk of cervical cancer)? ☐ ☐
- Does the client use sunscreen or wear protective clothing outdoors? ☐ ☐
- Does the client use safety equipment (eg, seat belts, hearing protection)? ☐ ☐
- Does the client engage in recreational activities that increase the risk of chronic health problems? ☐ ☐

HEALTH SYSTEM DIMENSION

- Does the client receive routine screening for chronic health problems? ☐ ☐
- Has the client been educated regarding risk factors for chronic health problems? ☐ ☐
- Does the client comply with treatment recommendations for conditions that increase the risk of chronic health problems? ☐ ☐
- Does the client take medications that increase the risk of accidental injury? ☐ ☐

▶ CHRONIC DISEASE RISK FACTOR MODIFICATION STRATEGIES

RISK FACTOR	STRATEGIES FOR MODIFICATION
Biophysical Dimension	
Presence of existing disease	Treat or control existing disease (eg, treat hypertension to decrease risk of heart disease)
Physical limitations	Caution against driving, other dangerous activity
Overweight	Encourage weight loss
Psychological Dimension	
Stress	Reduce stress levels if possible, teach coping skills
Physical Dimension	
Environmental pollutants	Advise to purify water, remain indoors on smoggy days, increase outside air exchange, replace asbestos insulation
Safety hazards	Eliminate safety hazards from home environment and neighborhood
Noise	Decrease noise level, encourage use of hearing protection
Temperature extremes	Maintain hydration, encourage appropriate clothing
Social Dimension	
Peer pressure	Teach coping skills, assertiveness
Social mores	Change societal attitudes to unhealthful behaviors
Occupational risk	Promote preventive measures (eg, safety precautions)
Behavioral Dimension	
Poor diet	Encourage well-balanced diet, educate on nutritional needs, assist with food budget, if needed
Substance abuse	Refer for treatment, if desired
Unsafe sexual activity	Encourage safer sexual practices, use of barrier contraceptives, limiting number of sexual partners, partner selectivity

RISK FACTOR	STRATEGIES FOR MODIFICATION
Behavioral Dimension	
Smoking	Encourage cessation, refer to cessation programs
Poor self-care practices	Encourage BSE/TSE on a regular basis
Sedentary lifestyle	Encourage physical activity
Sun exposure	Encourage use of sunscreen, protective clothing
High-risk recreation	Encourage use of appropriate equipment, safety practices
Health System Dimension	
Lack of routine screening	Refer for or provide screening for chronic diseases
Noncompliance	Encourage compliance with treatment regimens for conditions that increase the risk of chronic health problems

▶ SUBSTANCE ABUSE

Most drugs are used appropriately for medicinal purposes, but substance abuse is a growing world problem. The fact that many substances with the potential for abuse also have legitimate uses has made control of substance abuse difficult.

Because community health nurses interact with people in their homes, where most substance abuse occurs, they are in a unique position to identify persons with substance abuse problems. Community health nurses assess individuals, families, and communities for risk factors that may contribute to substance abuse, and they engage in primary prevention efforts to eliminate risk factors. Nurses assess individuals and families for signs of problems related to substance abuse and refer clients for assistance. They also provide support to individuals and families in dealing with problems of substance abuse.

At the community level, community health nurses may be engaged in political activities to modify risk factors that contribute to substance abuse. In addition, they may educate individuals and their families, as well as groups of clients, on the hazards of substance use and abuse in an effort to prevent or minimize these practices. See *Nursing in the Community: Dimensions of Community Health Nursing* (Chapter 33) for a full discussion of the role of the community health nurse with respect to substance abuse.

FETAL, NEONATAL, AND DEVELOPMENTAL EFFECTS OF PERINATAL PSYCHOACTIVE SUBSTANCE EXPOSURE

SUBSTANCE	FETAL EFFECTS	NEONATAL EFFECTS	DEVELOPMENTAL EFFECTS
Alcohol	Growth deficiency, microcephaly, stillbirth, low-birth weight (LBW), joint and facial anomalies, cardiac and kidney anomalies	Acute withdrawal with sedation, seizures, poor feeding	Developmental delay, low IQ, hyperactivity
Sedatives, hypnotics	Sedation at delivery	Tremors, hypertonicity poor suck, high-pitched cry	Unknown
Opioids	Intrauterine growth retardation, prematurity, microcephaly, hyperactivity	Withdrawal with tremors, hypertoxicity, poor feeding, diarrhea, seizures, irritability	Increased rate of sudden infant death syndrome (SIDS)
Cocaine	Spontaneous abortion	Tremors, hypertonicity, muscle weakness, seizures	Developmental delay, increased rate of SIDS
Amphetamines	Intrauterine growth retardation, biliary atresia, transposition of great vessels	Stillbirth, LBW, cardiac anomalies, withdrawal	Poor school performance
Hallucinogens	Agitation at delivery, microcephaly	Irritability, poor fine motor coordination, sensory input problems	Unknown
Cannabis	Bleeding problems in delivery	Sedation, tremors, excessive response to light	Unknown
Inhalants	Unknown	Unknown	Unknown
Nicotine	Intrauterine growth retardation, microcephaly	Jitteriness, poor feeding	Poor school performance, increased rate of SIDS

▶ SIGNS OF INTOXICATION WITH SELECTED PSYCHOACTIVE SUBSTANCES

SUBSTANCE	TYPICAL INDICATIONS OF INTOXICATION
Alcohol	Decreased alertness, impaired judgment, slurred speech, nausea, double vision, vertigo, staggering, unpredictable emotional changes, stupor, unconsciousness, increased reaction time
Sedatives, hypnotics, anxiolytics	Slurred speech, slow, shallow respirations, cold and clammy skin, nystagmus, weak and rapid pulse, drowsiness, blurred vision, unconsciousness, disorientation, depression, poor judgment, motor impairment
Opioids	Sedation, hypertension, respiratory depression, impaired intellectual function, constipation, pupillary constriction, watery eyes, increased pulse and blood pressure
Cocaine	Irritability, anxiety, slow weak pulse, slow, shallow breathing, sweating, dilated pupils, increased blood pressure, insomnia, seizures, dysinhibition, impulsivity, compulsive actions, hypersexuality, hypervigilance, hyperactivity
Amphetamines	Sweating, dilated pupils, increased blood pressure, agitation, fever, irritability, headache, chills, insomnia, agitation, tremors, seizures, wakefulness, hyperactivity, confusion, paranoia
Hallucinogens	Dilated pupils, mood swings, elevated blood pressure, paranoia, bizarre behavior, nausea and vomiting, tremors, panic, flushing, fever, sweating, agitation, aggression, nystagmus (PCP)
Cannabis	Reddened eyes, increased pulse, respirations, and blood pressure, laughter, confusion, panic, drowsiness
Inhalants	Giddiness, drowsiness, increased vital signs, headache, nausea, fainting, stupor, fatigue, slurred speech, disorientation, delirium
Nicotine	Headache, loss of appetite, nausea, increased pulse, blood pressure, and muscle tone

▶ INDICATIONS OF WITHDRAWAL FROM SELECTED PSYCHOACTIVE SUBSTANCES

SUBSTANCE	INDICATIONS OF WITHDRAWAL
Alcohol	Anxiety, insomnia, tremors, delirium, convulsions
Sedatives, hypnotics, anxiolytics	Anxiety, insomnia, tremors, delirium, convulsions (may occur up to 2 weeks after stopping use of anxiolytics)
Opioids	Restlessness, irritability, tremors, loss of appetite, panic, chills, sweating, cramps, watery eyes, runny nose, nausea, vomiting, muscle spasms, impaired coordination, depressed reflexes, dilated pupils, yawning
Cocaine	*Early crash:* agitation depression, anorexia, high level of craving, suicidal ideation *Middle crash:* fatigue, depression, no craving, insomnia *Late crash:* exhaustion, hypersomnolence, hyperphagia, no craving *Early withdrawal:* normal sleep and mood, low craving, low anxiety *Middle and late withdrawal:* anhedonia, anxiety, anergy, high level of craving exacerbated by conditioned cues *Extinction:* normal hedonic response and mood, episodic craving triggered by conditioned cues
Amphetamines	Fatigue, hunger, long periods of sleep, disorientation, severe depression
Hallucinogens	Slight irritability, restlessness, insomnia, reduced energy level, depression
Cannabis	Insomnia, hyperactivity, decreased appetite
Inhalants	None reported
Nicotine	Nervousness, increased appetite, sleep disturbances, anxiety, irritability

▶ SUBSTANCE ABUSE RISK FACTOR INVENTORY

Description: This inventory is intended to assist the community health nurse to identify clients at risk for substance abuse. Risk factors in the biophysical, psychological, social, behavioral, and health systems dimensions of health are addressed.

Appropriate populations: May be used with individual clients or population groups to identify risk factors amenable to modification. Appropriate to all age groups and cultural groups.

Data sources and data collection strategies: For individual clients, most of the information addressed in the inventory will be obtained from interviews with the client or significant others. Some information may also be available in existing health records. Information related to population groups will come from a variety of sources including local police and insurance statistics and records of local health care providers. Additional information may be obtained in interviews with or surveys of community residents or major informants such as health care providers, community officials, and so on.

Use of information: Risk factors identified in the use of the inventory provide a starting point for client education and efforts to modify risk factors to prevent the occurrence of substance abuse. Risk factor information may also be used to design community programs to prevent substance abuse.

▶ SUBSTANCE ABUSE RISK FACTOR INVENTORY

(Note: The "client" may be an individual or a group of people)   **YES**   **NO**

BIOPHYSICAL DIMENSION

- Is the client (population) in an age group at particular risk for substance abuse? ☐ ☐
- Does the client have a family history of substance abuse? ☐ ☐
- Does the client have an existing physical condition that might lead to substance abuse? ☐ ☐
- Does the client exhibit periodic signs of intoxication? ☐ ☐
- Does the client exhibit periodic signs of withdrawal? ☐ ☐
- Does the client exhibit signs and symptoms of long-term effects of substance abuse? ☐ ☐
- Is the client pregnant? ☐ ☐
- Does the client have a history of fetal exposure to addictive substances? ☐ ☐
- Does the client have difficulty sleeping? ☐ ☐

PSYCHOLOGICAL DIMENSION   YES   NO

- Is the client under stress? ☐ ☐
- Does the client have a poor self-image? ☐ ☐
- Does the client have realistic life goals? ☐ ☐
- Does the client exhibit poor impulse control? ☐ ☐
- Does the client have poor coping skills? ☐ ☐
- Is the client depressed?
- Has the client experienced a recent significant loss? ☐ ☐
- Does the client have a history of mental or emotional illness? ☐ ☐
- Does the client currently exhibit signs of other psychopathology? ☐ ☐

SOCIAL DIMENSION

- Do community norms support substance abuse? ☐ ☐
- Do the client's peers support substance abuse? ☐ ☐
- Is alcohol or drug use a regular part of social interaction? ☐ ☐
- Are drugs and alcohol easily accessible? ☐ ☐
- Is legislation regarding drug and alcohol access enforced? ☐ ☐
- Do cultural or religious values influence drug or alcohol use? ☐ ☐
- Is the client unemployed? ☐ ☐
- Is the client experiencing financial difficulties? ☐ ☐

SOCIAL DIMENSION | YES | NO

- Is the client subjected to discrimination? ☐ ☐
- Do occupational factors increase the client's risk of substance abuse? ☐ ☐
- Does the client have a history of frequent work or school absence? ☐ ☐
- Has the client had difficulty meeting work or school expectations? ☐ ☐
- Is the client experiencing difficulty in interpersonal interactions? ☐ ☐
- Is the client experiencing difficulty in family interactions? ☐ ☐
- Has the client been a victim of family violence? ☐ ☐
- Does the client engage in violent behavior? ☐ ☐
- Is the client socially isolated? ☐ ☐
- Is the client homeless? ☐ ☐
- Is the client engaged in criminal activity related to drugs or alcohol? ☐ ☐

BEHAVIORAL DIMENSION

- Does the client report a loss of appetite? ☐ ☐
- Does the client smoke? ☐ ☐
- Does the client use drugs recreationally? ☐ ☐
- Is drug or alcohol use associated with leisure activities? ☐ ☐
- Does the client engage in other high-risk behaviors (eg, driving while intoxicated)? ☐ ☐
- Does the client engage in prostitution for drugs? ☐ ☐

HEALTH SYSTEM DIMENSION

- Has the client received prescriptions for psychoactive drugs? ☐ ☐
- Does the client have a history of past substance abuse treatment? ☐ ☐

► SUBSTANCE ABUSE RISK FACTOR MODIFICATION STRATEGIES

RISK FACTOR	STRATEGIES FOR MODIFICATION
Biophysical Dimension	
Presence of existing disease	Treat or control existing disease, assist client to adjust to disease or disability, refer for counseling if needed
Pregnancy	Caution against drug and alcohol use during pregnancy
Insomnia	Refer for assistance, counseling as needed
Psychological Dimension	
Stress	Reduce stress levels if possible, teach coping skills
Poor self-image	Enhance self-image, refer for counseling as needed
Poor impulse control	Refer for counseling
Depression	Refer for therapy, medication as needed
Recent loss	Assist with grieving, refer to support groups, counseling
Mental illness	Refer for treatment
Unrealistic expectations	Encourage more realistic expectations by client and others
Social Dimension	
Peer pressure	Teach coping skills, assertiveness
Social mores	Change societal attitudes to unhealthful behaviors
Easy access	Political action for legislation and enforcement limiting access, encourage adequate supervision of children and adolescents
Discrimination	Political advocacy
Unemployment, homelessness	Refer for financial assistance, employment, housing
Family interactions	Refer for counseling, teach good communication skills
Family violence	Remove from home, refer to protective services, refer for counseling
Social isolation	Encourage development of social network, refer to community support groups

RISK FACTOR	STRATEGIES FOR MODIFICATION
Behavioral Dimension	
Prostitution	Discourage prostitution for drugs, encourage safe sexual practices
Smoking	Encourage cessation, refer to cessation programs
Leisure activity	Encourage non-drug- and alcohol-related leisure activities
Other risk behaviors	Discourage driving or other dangerous activity while intoxicated
Health System Dimension	
Prescription drugs	Caution against abuse of prescription drugs, report providers who overprescribe controlled substances

▶ TREATMENT MODALITIES TYPICALLY USED FOR SELECTED FORMS OF PSYCHOACTIVE SUBSTANCE ABUSE

SUBSTANCE	TYPICAL TREATMENT MODALITIES
Alcohol	Detoxification; psychotherapy; group therapy; family therapy; self-help groups (Alcoholics Anonymous, Al-Anon); pharmacologic therapy (disulfiram, short-term use of tranquilizers or antidepressants); residential programs; referral for vocational rehabilitation and social services as needed
Sedatives, hypnotics, anxiolytics	Detoxification; psychotherapy and group therapy (for underlying psychiatric disorders)
Opioids	Pharmacologic therapy (methadone, opioid antagonists); therapeutic communities (Synanon, Odyssey House, Daytop, Phoenix House); group therapy; assistance with social skills, vocational training and job placement; family therapy; self-help groups (Narcotics Anonymous, Chemical Dependency Anonymous); psychotherapy
Cocaine	Hospitalization; self-help groups; contingency contracting (client agreement to urinary monitoring and acceptance of aversive contingencies for positive results); pharmacologic therapy (tricyclic antidepressants)

Amphetamines	No established treatment guidelines; may be similar to treatment for cocaine abuse
Hallucinogens	Detoxification; psychotherapy (for underlying psychiatric disorders); group therapy; residential programs
Cannabis	Same as for Hallucinogens; self-help groups
Inhalants	Psychosocial interventions; psychotherapy (for underlying psychiatric disorder); sociodrama; vocational rehabilitation; family therapy; social support services
Nicotine	Aversive conditioning; desensitization; substitution; hypnotherapy; group therapy; relaxation training; supportive therapy; abrupt abstinence

▶ VIOLENCE

Violence is a pervasive phenomenon in U.S. society. In part, this is a function of the U.S. heritage and the activities required to carve a nation from a wild and uncivilized land. Violence has historically been seen as a mode of resolving conflict and even of ensuring support of law and order. The vigilante approach to justice on the Western frontier is one example of the use of violence to protect society.

In societies in which survival is subject to physical threats that must be countered by physical force, violent behavior may be more or less of a necessity. Some authorities, however, contend that humankind has failed to adapt to changes in survival needs and has continued to exercise proclivities to violence that are not warranted in today's society.

Family violence, homicide, and suicide are forms of violence that are of particular concern to society, and, hence, to community health nurses who are charged with promoting the health of the population. Violence contributes to a variety of physical and psychological health problems that can be prevented by community health nursing efforts to modify factors that contribute to violence against self or others. See *Nursing in the Community: Dimensions of Community Health Nursing* (Chapter 34) for an in-depth discussion of violence as a community health problem.

▶ PHYSICAL AND PSYCHOLOGICAL INDICATIONS OF CHILD ABUSE

TYPE OF ABUSE	PHYSICAL INDICATIONS	PSYCHOLOGICAL INDICATIONS
Neglect	Persistent hunger Poor hygiene Inappropriate dress for the weather Constant fatigue Unattended physical health problems Poor growth patterns	Delinquency due to lack of supervision School truancy Begging or stealing food
Physical abuse	Bruises or welts in unusual places or in several stages of healing; distinctive shapes Burns (especially cigarette burns; immersion burns of hands, feet, or buttocks; rope burns; or distinctively shaped burns)	Wary of physical contact with adults Apprehensive when other children cry Behavioral extremes of withdrawal or aggression Appears frightened of parents

TYPE OF ABUSE	PHYSICAL INDICATIONS	PSYCHOLOGICAL INDICATIONS
	Fractures (multiple or in various stages of healing, inconsistent with explanations of injury)	Inappropriate response to pain
	Joint swelling or limited mobility	
	Long-bone deformities	
	Lacerations and abrasions to the mouth, lip, gums, eye, genitalia	
	Human bite marks	
	Signs of intracranial trauma	
	Deformed or displaced nasal septum	
	Bleeding or fluid drainage from the ears or ruptured eardrums	
	Broken, loose, or missing teeth	
	Difficulty in respirations, tenderness or crepitus over ribs	
	Abdominal pain or tenderness	
	Recurrent urinary tract infection	
Emotional abuse	Nothing specific	Overly compliant, passive, and undemanding
		Extremely aggressive, demanding, or angry
		Behavior inappropriate for age (either overly adult or overly infantile)
		Developmental delay
		Attempted suicide
Sexual abuse	Torn, stained, or bloody underwear	Withdrawn
	Pain or itching in genital areas	Engages in fantasy or infantile behavior
	Bruises or bleeding from external genitalia, vagina, rectum	Poor peer relationships
		Unwilling to participate in physical activities

TYPE OF ABUSE	PHYSICAL INDICATIONS	PSYCHOLOGICAL INDICATIONS
	Sexually transmitted disease	Wears long sleeves and several layers of clothes even in hot weather
	Swollen or red cervix, vulva, or perineum	
	Semen around the mouth or genitalia or on clothing	Delinquency or running away
	Pregnancy	Inappropriate sexual behavior or mannerisms

▶ PHYSICAL AND PSYCHOLOGICAL INDICATIONS OF SPOUSE ABUSE

PHYSICAL INDICATIONS	PSYCHOLOGICAL INDICATIONS
Chronic fatigue	Casual response to a serious injury or excessively emotional response to a relatively minor injury
Vague complaints, aches, and pains	
Frequent injuries	Frequent ambulatory or emergency room visits
Recurrent sexually transmitted diseases	Nightmares
	Depression
Muscle tension	Anxiety
Facial lacerations	Anorexia or other eating disorder
Injuries to chest, breasts, back, abdomen, or genitalia	Drug or alcohol abuse
	Poor self-esteem
Bilateral injuries of arms or legs	Suicide attempts
Symmetric injuries	
Obvious patterns of belt buckles, bite marks, fist or hand marks	
Burns of hands, feet, buttocks, or with distinctive patterns	
Headaches	
Ulcers	

▶ PHYSICAL AND PSYCHOLOGICAL INDICATIONS OF ELDER ABUSE

TYPE OF ABUSE	PHYSICAL INDICATIONS	PSYCHOLOGICAL INDICATIONS
Neglect	Constant hunger or malnutrition	Listlessness
		Social isolation

TYPE OF ABUSE	PHYSICAL INDICATIONS	PSYCHOLOGICAL INDICATIONS
	Poor hygiene	
	Inappropriate dress for the weather	
	Chronic fatigue	
	Unattended medical needs	
	Poor skin integrity or decubiti	
	Contractures	
	Urine burns/excoriation	
	Dehydration	
	Fecal impaction	
Emotional abuse	Hypochondria	Habit disorder (biting, sucking, rocking)
		Destructive or antisocial conduct
		Neurotic traits (sleep or speech disorder, inhibition of play)
		Hysteria
		Obsessions or compulsions
		Phobias
Physical abuse	Bruises and welts	Withdrawal
	Burns	Confusion
	Fractures	Fear of caretaker or other family members
	Sprains or dislocations	
	Lacerations or abrasions	Listlessness
	Evidence of oversedation	
Sexual abuse	Difficulty walking	Withdrawal
	Torn, stained, or bloody underwear	
	Pain or itching in genital area	
	Bruises or bleeding on external genitalia or in vaginal or anal areas	
	Sexually transmitted diseases	
Financial abuse	Inappropriate clothing	Failure to meet financial obligations
	Unmet medical needs	Anxiety over expenses
Denial of rights	Nothing specific	Hesitancy in making decisions
		Listlessness and apathy

▶ ADVANTAGES AND DISADVANTAGES OF FINANCIAL ARRANGEMENTS TO PREVENT FINANCIAL ABUSE OF THE ELDERLY

TYPE OF FINANCIAL ARRANGEMENT	ADVANTAGES	DISADVANTAGES
Financial representative trust	Legal accountability for use of funds Ability to specify use of funds and beneficiaries	Cost of establishing and administering trust
Durable power of attorney	Financial needs met if older person becomes incapacitated Ability to designate person to control funds Retention of control of funds by older person until he or she chooses to relinquish it or becomes incapacitated	Limited measures to safeguard older person if designee does not use funds as intended
Representative payee	Limited control of funds by designated payee Legal responsibility to use funds for the benefit of the stated beneficiary Mechanism for demanding accounting of use of funds	Restrictions on types of funds covered
Joint tenancy	Ability of older person to designate recipient of funds Automatic right of survivorship eliminates inheritance taxes	Both parties have access to and use of property and the joint tenant may use them for his or her own benefit and not that of the older person

▶ FAMILY VIOLENCE RISK FACTOR INVENTORY

Description: This inventory is intended to assist the community health nurse to identify clients at risk for family violence. The inventory assesses risk for all forms of family violence, including child abuse, spouse abuse, and elder abuse. Risk factors in the biophysical, psychological, social, behavioral and health system dimensions of health are addressed.

Appropriate populations: May be used with individual clients or population groups to identify risk factors amenable to modification. Appropriate to all age groups and cultural groups.

Data sources and data collection strategies: For individual clients, most of the information addressed in the inventory will be obtained from interviews with the client or significant others. Some information may also be available in existing health or protective services records. Information related to population groups will come from a variety of sources including local police and health agency records and news releases. Additional information may be obtained in interviews with or surveys of community residents or major informants such as health care providers, community officials, and so on.

Use of information: Risk factors identified in the use of the inventory provide a starting point for client and community education and efforts to modify risk factors to prevent the occurrence of family violence. Risk factor information may also be used to design community programs to prevent violence.

▶ FAMILY VIOLENCE RISK FACTOR INVENTORY

(Note: The "client" may be an individual or a group of people)	YES	NO

BIOPHYSICAL DIMENSION

	YES	NO
• Are family members in age groups at particular risk for abuse?	☐	☐
• Do family members have existing physical conditions that increase the risk of violence?	☐	☐
• Is there physical evidence of neglect or abuse in family members?	☐	☐
• Is a member of the family pregnant?	☐	☐
• Is there a history of head trauma in a family member?	☐	☐

PSYCHOLOGICAL DIMENSION

	YES	NO
• Are family members under stress?	☐	☐
• Do family members have poor self-concepts?	☐	☐
• Do family members have poor coping skills?	☐	☐
• Do family members exhibit poor impulse control?	☐	☐
• Are family members depressed?		
• Is there a negative emotional climate in the family?	☐	☐
• Is there a family history of mental or emotional illness?	☐	☐
• Do family members exhibit annoying traits?	☐	☐
• Are expectations of family members unrealistic?	☐	☐
• Do some family members have excessive power over others?	☐	☐

SOCIAL DIMENSION

	YES	NO
• Do community norms support family violence?	☐	☐
• Do significant others support family violence?	☐	☐
• Have family members been subject to past abuse?	☐	☐
• Are family interactions positive?	☐	☐
• Is the family experiencing financial difficulty?	☐	☐
• Do cultural or religious values influence the risk of violence?	☐	☐
• Is one or more family members unemployed?	☐	☐
• Is the family socially isolated?	☐	☐
• Does the family have an inadequate social support network?	☐	☐
• Is there evidence of emotional or economic dependence among family members?	☐	☐

BEHAVIORAL DIMENSION	YES	NO
• Do family members use or abuse alcohol?	☐	☐
• Do family members use or abuse drugs?	☐	☐
• Is one family member excessively sexually dominant?	☐	☐
• Is cohabitation present in the family?	☐	☐

HEALTH SYSTEM DIMENSION		
• Do family members make frequent use of health services (especially emergency services)?	☐	☐
• Do family members have a regular source of health care?	☐	☐
• Do health or medical care needs create stress for family members?	☐	☐

▶ FAMILY VIOLENCE RISK FACTOR MODIFICATION STRATEGIES

RISK FACTOR	STRATEGIES FOR MODIFICATION
Biophysical Dimension	
Presence of existing disease	Treat or control existing disease, assist client and family to adjust to disease or disability, refer for counseling if needed, provide respite
Pregnancy	Refer for prenatal care, assess family attitudes to pregnancy, refer for counseling as needed
Head trauma	Refer for medication, rehabilitation, counseling as needed
Psychological Dimension	
Stress	Reduce stress levels if possible, teach coping skills
Poor self-image	Enhance self-image, refer for counseling as needed
Poor impulse control	Refer for counseling
Depression	Refer for therapy, medication as needed
Mental illness	Refer for treatment
Unrealistic expectations	Encourage more realistic expectations by client and others
Negative emotional climate	Encourage expression of positive emotions, teach effective communication skills
Annoying behaviors/traits	Assist family members to change behaviors or reframe perceptions or responses to annoying behaviors, teach coping skills, teach assertiveness
Power allocation	Assist family to renegotiate power structure
Social Dimension	
Social mores	Change societal attitudes to violence
Unemployment, homelessness	Refer for financial assistance, employment, housing
Family interactions	Refer for counseling, teach good communication skills
Social isolation	Encourage development of social network, refer to community support groups

RISK FACTOR	STRATEGIES FOR MODIFICATION
Social Dimension	
Emotional or economic dependence	Refer for assistance in developing independence, support independence
Past exposure to abuse	Refer for counseling, role model effective interactions
Behavioral Dimension	
Substance use or abuse	Refer for treatment, refer to individual and family support groups
Cohabitation	Encourage realistic assessment of risk for violence
Sexual domination	Refer for counseling, teach assertiveness
Health System Dimension	
Lack of regular health care	Refer for regular source of health care
Stressful health care needs	Coordinate health-related activities, provide respite as needed, refer for financial assistance as needed

▶ SUICIDE RISK FACTOR INVENTORY

Description: This inventory is intended to assist the community health nurse to identify clients at risk for suicide. Risk factors in each of the six dimensions of health are addressed.

Appropriate populations: May be used with individual clients or population groups to identify risk factors amenable to modification. Appropriate to all age groups and cultural groups.

Data sources and data collection strategies: For individual clients, most of the information addressed in the inventory will be obtained from interviews with the client or significant others. Some information may also be available in existing health records. Information related to population groups will come from a variety of sources including local police and insurance statistics and records of local health care providers. Additional information may be obtained in interviews with or surveys of community residents or major informants such as health care providers, community officials, and so on.

Use of information: Risk factors identified in the use of the inventory enable the community health nurse to initiate interventions to prevent suicide by individual clients. Risk factor information may also be used to design community programs to prevent suicide.

▶ SUICIDE RISK FACTOR INVENTORY

(Note: The "client" may be an individual or a group of people)	YES	NO

BIOPHYSICAL DIMENSION

- Is the client (population) in an age group at particular risk for suicide? ☐ ☐
- Does the client have an existing physical condition that might lead to suicide? ☐ ☐
- Is the client experiencing a developmental or maturational crisis (eg, adolescence)? ☐ ☐
- Is the client experiencing significant pain? ☐ ☐
- Does the client report insomnia? ☐ ☐

PSYCHOLOGICAL DIMENSION

- Is the client under stress? ☐ ☐
- Does the client have poor coping skills? ☐ ☐
- Does the client have a poor self-concept? ☐ ☐
- Does the client have unrealistic expectations of self? ☐ ☐
- Has the client recently experienced what he or she perceives as a failure? ☐ ☐
- Is the client depressed? ☐ ☐
- Has the client experienced a recent significant loss? ☐ ☐
- Does the client have a history of mental or emotional illness? ☐ ☐
- Has the client expressed feelings of hopelessness or despair? ☐ ☐
- Has the client expressed suicidal thoughts or intentions? ☐ ☐
- Does the client describe specific plans for suicide? ☐ ☐
- Has the client made a previous suicide attempt? ☐ ☐

PHYSICAL DIMENSION

- Does the client experience seasonal affective disorder? ☐ ☐

SOCIAL DIMENSION

- Has a friend or family member attempted or completed suicide? ☐ ☐
- Has the client been exposed to suicide or a suicide attempt by others (*personally or via media coverage*)? ☐ ☐
- Has the client been a victim of abuse? ☐ ☐
- Is the client experiencing family or interpersonal difficulties? ☐ ☐

SOCIAL DIMENSION	YES	NO
• Has the client exhibited poor work or school performance?	☐	☐
• Does the client have easy access to lethal methods of suicide?	☐	☐
• Is the client unemployed?	☐	☐
• Is the client experiencing financial difficulties?	☐	☐
• Is the client socially isolated?	☐	☐
• Is the client homeless?	☐	☐

BEHAVIORAL DIMENSION	YES	NO
• Does the client report a loss of appetite?	☐	☐
• Does the client abuse alcohol or drugs?	☐	☐
• Does the client engage in regular exercise?	☐	☐
• Does the client have any leisure activities?	☐	☐

HEALTH SYSTEM DIMENSION

• Does the client have a regular source of health care?	☐	☐

▶ SUICIDE RISK FACTOR MODIFICATION STRATEGIES

RISK FACTOR	STRATEGIES FOR MODIFICATION
Biophysical Dimension	
Presence of existing disease	Treat or control existing disease, assist client and family to adjust to disease or disability, refer for counseling if needed, provide respite
Pain	Provide pain medication, suggest alternative therapies for pain control (eg, acupuncture, relaxation therapy), refer for pain management
Insomnia	Refer for assistance
Psychological Dimension	
Stress	Reduce stress levels if possible, teach coping skills
Poor self-image	Enhance self-image, refer for counseling as needed
Depression	Refer for therapy, medication as needed
Mental illness	Refer for treatment
Unrealistic expectations	Encourage more realistic expectations by client and others
Social Dimension	
Social mores	Change societal attitudes to violence
Unemployment, homelessness	Refer for financial assistance, employment, housing
Family interactions	Refer for counseling, teach good communication skills
Social isolation	Encourage development of social network, refer to community support groups
Past exposure to abuse	Refer for counseling, role model effective interactions
Behavioral Dimension	
Substance use or abuse	Refer for treatment, refer to individual and family support groups
Lack of exercise	Encourage regular physical activity
Lack of leisure activity	Encourage enjoyable leisure activity
Health System Dimension	
Lack of regular health care	Refer for regular source of health care

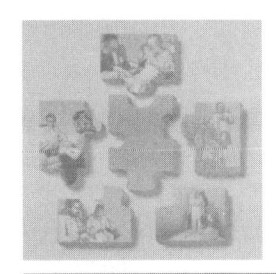

INDEX

A

Abortion. *See* Spontaneous abortion
Abuse. *See also* Child abuse; Spouse abuse; Violence
 in older clients, prevention for, 133
 prior exposure to, and family violence, 243
Accommodation, in group development, 41
Acne, 160
Acquired immune deficiency syndrome (AIDS), 160
Acute health problems, in school setting, 160
 tertiary prevention for, 172
Acyclovir, for herpes simplex virus, 208
Adolescents
 developmental characteristics of, 89–90
 Health Assessment Guide for, 92
 home safety inventory for, 23

Adult(s)
 developmental characteristics of, 89–90
 immunization recommendations for, 67–68
Adult clients, 89–109
 Health Assessment Guide for, 92–100
Advanced activities of daily living, 119
Advocate, community health nurse role as, 218
African Americans, children, screening for sickle cell disease, 67
Aging
 common physical changes of, implications for health, 110–113
 myths about, 110
Air pollution, primary preventive measures for, 55–56
Airborne transmission, of communicable diseases, portals of entry and exit for, 204
Al-Anon, 232
Alcohol, 10, 225–227

249

Alcohol abuse, 134, 232
Alcoholics Anonymous, 232
Allergic dermatitis, 86
Alpha-interferon, for Hepatitis C, 207
Amantadine, for influenza, 209
Amoxicillin, for Lyme disease, 209
Amphetamines, 225–227, 233
Amphotericin B, for coccidioidomycosis, 205
Anemia, in school setting, 160
Anger, and discipline, 70
Animal bites, 204, 217
Animals, primary preventive measures for, 54–55
Annoying behaviors, and family violence, 242
Anorexia, 10
Antacids, 10
Anthropological literature, 45
Anthropometric measurements, 4
Antibiotics, 10
Anticipatory guidance, 64–66, 84
Anticoagulants, 10
Anticonvulsants, 10
Antidepressants, 10, 232
Antihypertensives, 10
Antimony, as occupational hazard, 174
Antineoplastics, 10
Antituberculins, 10, 212
Antiviral agents, for HIV, 208
Anxiolytics, 226–227, 232
Appearance, and personal safety considerations, in home visiting, 18–19
Appetite, decreased, in children, anticipatory guidance for, 65
Arsenic, as occupational hazard, 174
Arthritis, in school setting, 160
Asbestos, as occupational hazard, 173
Asphyxiation, health hazards and, 174
Aspirin, 10
Asthma, 160, 174
Asymmetrical tonic neck reflex, 68
Attention deficit hyperactivity disorder, 160
Attention span, assessment of, 121
Aversion conditioning, 233
Azithromycin, for chlamydia, 204

B

Babinski sign, 72
Bacterial conjunctivitis, school readmission guidelines for, 160
Basic activities of daily living, 117–118
Bedtime resistance, 66, 88
Bedwetting, in children, 86
Behavioral data, in health education process, 12
Behavioral dimension, 2
Behaviors, annoying, as risk factor in family violence, 242
Beta-globulin, normal values for, 114
Biliary atresia, 225
Biophysical dimension, 2
Birth history, 72
Births, assessment of, 152
Blindness, 160
Blood, health hazards and, 174
Blood pressure, screening in children, 67
Blood tests, normal values for, 114
Blood urea nitrogen (BUN), normal values for, 114
Bloodborne diseases, universal precautions for, 19–20

INDEX

Body systems
  aging and, implications for health in, 110–113
  health problems with, in school setting, 160
  review of, 26–28, 76–77, 90, 93–94, 124–125
Bordetella pertussis, 210. *See also* Pertussis
Borrelia burgdorferi, 209. *See also* Lyme disease
Breast self-examination (BSE), 107–108
Burns, health hazards and, 174

C

Cadmium, as occupational hazard, 174
Cancer, 160, 175
Cannabis, 225–227, 233
Cardiovascular system
  aging and, implications for health in, 111
  health hazards and, 174
  health problems with, in school setting, 160
Caregiver, community health nurse role as, 218
Caretaker, stress on, assessment of, 91
Case management process, 2, 31–32
Case manager, community health nurse role as, 218
Cathartics, 10
Ceftriaxone, for gonorrhea, 205
Central nervous system, 160, 174
Cerebral palsy, in school setting, 160
Change process, 2
Chemical Dependency Anonymous, 232

Chickenpox
  school readmission guidelines for, 160
  in school setting, 160
Child abuse
  evidence of, in assessment of children, 73
  physical and psychological indications of, 234–235
  risk factors for, 239
  suspected, nursing interventions for, 87
Child care, and communicable disease, 217
Child development, anticipatory guidance for, 64–66
Child Health Assessment Guide, 75–83
Children. *See also* Schoolchildren; *specific ages groups*
  assessment of
    Denver II and, 72, 75
    general considerations in, 72–73
    variations in physical findings in, 72
  as clients, 61–88
  common health problems in, nursing interventions for, 85–88
  developmental characteristics of, 62–63
  disciplining of, 70–71
  home safety inventory for, 21–23
  immunization recommendations for, 67–68
  nutritional status of, questions for assessment of, 73–74
  physical examination of
    pace of, 72
    respecting physical modesty in, 72
    restraining in, 72

Children (*cont.*)
  primary prevention interventions for, 84
  routine screening for, 67
  with special needs, parental assistance for, 84
Chlamydia, 204
Chlamydia trachomatis, 204
Cholesterol, normal values for, 114
Chronic Disease Risk Factor Inventory, 219–221
Chronic health problems, 218–223
  clients with
    community health nurse's roles and, 218
    functional ability of. *See* Functional Health Status Inventory
  risk factor modification strategies for, 222–223
  in school setting, 160, 172
CK. *See* Creatinine kinase (CK)
Client(s). *See also* Adult clients; Children; Family, as client; Home health clients; Older clients
  characteristics of, and learning situation, 12
  maturation of, and health education process, 12
Client Discharge Inventory, 33–36
Climbing, in children, anticipatory guidance for, 65
Clostridium tetani, 212. *See also* Tetanus
Cocaine, 225–227, 232
Coccidioides immitis, 204
Coccidioidomycosis, 204–205
Cognitive dimension, 2
Cognitive Function Assessment Guide, 120–122
Cohabitation, and family violence, modification strategies for, 243

Cohabiting families, 135
Colic, in children, 85
Communal families, 135
Communicable disease(s), 203–218
  modes of transmission in, portals of entry and exit for, 204
  risk factor modification strategies for, 217–218
Communicable Disease Risk Factor Inventory, 213–216
Community(ies)
  environmental hazards for, primary preventive measures for, 53–56
  geopolitical, 152
  Health Assessment and Intervention Planning Guide for, 149–158
  substance abuse in, 224
Community agencies, and Resource File Entry Form, 37
Community assessment, 148
  data sources in, 148–149
Community Disaster Assessment and Planning Guide, 193–201
Community disaster potential, 199
Community Disaster Preparedness Checklist, 192
Community disaster response, stages of, 189–190
Community disaster warning signals, 191
Community health nurse
  political activities of, and substance abuse, 224
  roles of
    and chronic health problems, 218
    in disaster setting, 189
    in school setting, 161
    and substance abuse, 224

and violence issues, 234–237
in work setting, ethical issues of, 180
Community health nursing
Dimensions Model of. *See* Dimensions Model
in school setting, 170–172
Community resources, 37
Community Safety Inventory. *See* Neighborhood/Community Safety Inventory
Compliance, and discipline, 70–71
Concentration, assessment of, 121
Confidentiality, regarding employees health problems, in work setting, 180
Confusion, in older clients, secondary prevention for, 133
Conjunctivitis, bacterial, school readmission guidelines for, 160
Consistency, and discipline, 70
Constipation, 85, 132, 160
Constructed environment, safety hazards in, 58–59
Consultant, community health nurse as, 161
Consumption patterns, 96, 127, 140, 155, 165, 185
Contamination, of food or water, and communicable disease, 217
Content, selection and sequencing of, in health education process, 11
Contingency contracting, 232
Contraceptives, oral, 10
Cooking activities, assessment of, 118
Coordinator, community health nurse as, 161
Coping skills, 84, 170–171

Corynebacterium diphtheriae, 205. *See also* Diphtheria
Counseling, in school setting, 171
Counselor, community health nurse role as, 218
Cradle cap, in children, 86
Crawling, in children, anticipatory guidance for, 64
Creatinine, normal values for, 114
Creatinine kinase (CK), normal values for, 115
Creeping, in children, anticipatory guidance for, 64
Cultural Assessment Guide, 45–52
Cultural exploration, modes of, 44
Cultural influences
and assessment of men's health, 91
and Cognitive Function Assessment Guide, 120
on dimensions of health, 43–52
and health education process, 12
on women's health, 91
Culturally relevant care, 43–44
Cumulative trauma, as occupational hazard, 173

D

Daily diet history, 6–7
Data, in community assessment, 148–149
Daytop, 232
Deafness, 160
Death
leading causes of, in United States, 218
preparation for, in older clients, 132
Delayed speech, in children, 87
Delivery, bleeding problems in, 225

Dementia, clients with, functional ability of. *See* Functional Health Status Inventory
Denial of rights, of elderly, psychological indications of, 237
Dental care, in children
  primary preventive interventions for, 84
  screening of, 67
Dental caries, 160
Denver II, in assessment of children, 72, 75
Dependence, emotional or economic, and family violence, 243
Depression
  in older clients, 133
  as risk factor
    for communicable disease, 217
    in family violence, 242
    for substance abuse, 231
Dermatitis, 160, 174
Desensitization, 233
Detoxification, for substance abuse, 232–233
Development, in children, 84
Development history, 72
Developmental characteristics
  of adolescents, 89–90
  of adults, 89–90
  of children, 62–63
Developmental milestones, 72
Developmental tasks, in family development, 135–136
Diabetes mellitus, 160
Diaper rash, in children, 85–86
Diarrhea, 85, 160
Diet, poor, and chronic diseases, 222
Dietary history
  daily, 6–7
  and nutritional assessment, 4

Dimensions Model
  of community health nursing, 1–2
  components of, 2
  dimensions of health. *See* Dimensions of health
  dimensions of health care. *See* Dimensions of health care
  dimensions of nursing. *See* Dimensions of nursing
Dimensions of health
  components of, 2
  cultural influences on, 43–52
  environmental influences on, 52–56
  influences on, 43–60
Dimensions of health care, components of, 2
Dimensions of nursing, components of, 2
Diphtheria, 205
  immunizations for, 67, 205
  in older clients, 132
  school readmission guidelines for, 160
  in school setting, 160
Diphtheria, tetanus, pertussis vaccines (DPT)
  booster, for pertussis, 210
  recommendations for administration, 67
Diphtheria antitoxin, 205
Direct contact transmission, of communicable diseases, portals of entry and exit for, 204
Direct inoculation contact transmission, of communicable diseases, portals of entry and exit for, 204
Director, community health nurse as, 161
Disability, with chronic health problems, 218

INDEX 255

Disaster Assessment and Planning Guide, 193–201
  vulnerable populations in, 199
Disaster plan elements, 200–201
Disaster potential, 59
Disaster preparedness, client education related to, 191
Disaster prevention/mitigation activities, 200
Disaster response. *See* Community disaster response
Disaster setting, 189–201
Disaster warning signals, 191
Discharge. *See* Client Discharge Inventory
Discipline, principles of, 70–71
Discrimination, and substance abuse, modification strategies for, 231
Disease, emergence of, 203
Dissolution, in group development, 41
Disulfiram, for treatment of alcohol abuse, 232
Diuretics, 10
Documentation, in home visits, 20
Douching, and communicable disease, modification strategies for, 218
Doxycycline, 204–205, 209
DPT. *See* Diphtheria, tetanus, pertussis vaccines (DPT)
Dressing activities
  assessment of, 117
  in children, anticipatory guidance for, 66
Duodenal ulcer, 160
Durable power of attorney, advantages and disadvantages of, 238

Dust, as occupational hazard, 174
Dysmenorrhea, 160

E

Earthquakes, disaster preparedness for, 191
Economic dependence, and family violence, modification strategies for, 243
Eczema, 160
Education, health of schoolchildren and, 159
Educational assessment, 12–17
Educational literature, 45
Educational Planning and Implementation Guide, 12–17
Educator, community health nurse as, 218
  in school setting, 161
Elder abuse. *See also* Financial abuse
  physical and psychological indications of, 236–237
  risk factors for, 239
Electrical hazard, as occupational hazard, 174
Electrocution, health hazards and, 174
Emergency stage, 189–190
Emotional abuse, indications of
  in children, 235
  in elderly, 237
Emotional climate, negative, and family violence, modification strategies for, 242
Emotional dependence, and family violence, modification strategies for, 243

256　INDEX

Employees
　health problems of, and confidentiality in work setting, 180
　Work Fitness Inventory for, 176–179
Encopresis, 160
Endocrine system
　aging and, implications for health in, 113
　health problems with, in school setting, 160
Enuresis, 160
Environment, and Child Health Assessment Guide, 78–79
Environmental changes, and emergence of diseases, 203
Environmental influences, on dimensions of health, 52–56
Environmental pollutants, and chronic diseases, modification strategies for, 222
Epidemiologic process, 2
Erythromycin, 204–205, 210
Ethical dimension, 2
Ethical issues, in work setting, 180
Evacuation, disaster preparedness plans for, 191
Exclusion, from school, conditions typically warranting, 160–161
Exercise, in older clients, primary prevention strategies for, 132
Expectations, unrealistic
　and family violence, 242
　and substance abuse, 231
Exploration, in children, anticipatory guidance for, 64–65
Exposure, extreme weather, as occupational hazard, 174
Extended families, 135

F

Family(ies)
　as client, 135–158
　　Health Assessment and Intervention Planning Guide for, 137–144
　cohabiting, 135
　communal, 135
　environmental hazards for, 53–56
　extended, 135
　homosexual, 135
　nuclear conjugal, 135
　single-parent, 135
　stepfamilies, 135
　substance abuse in, 224
Family Crisis Assessment Guide, 145–147
Family development, stages of, 135–136
Family interactions
　and family violence, 242
　and substance abuse, 231
Family problems, effects of, in work setting, 180
Family roles, 139
Family therapy, for substance abuse, 232–233
Family violence
　risk factor modification strategies for, 242–243
　and substance abuse, 231
　and women, assessment for, 91
Family Violence Risk Factor Inventory, 239–241
Fatigue, and communicable disease, 217
Fecal-oral transmission, of communicable diseases, portals of entry and exit for, 204

Feeding activities
  assessment of, 117
  in children, anticipatory guidance for, 64
Feeding history, 72
Fetus, growth deficiency in, 225
Financial abuse
  financial arrangement to prevent, 238
  physical and psychological indications of, 237
Financial representative trust, 238
Financial resources, inadequate, in older clients, 134
Fire
  disaster preparedness for, 191
  as occupational hazard, 174
Fire escape ladders, 191
Floods, disaster preparedness for, 191
Fluconazole, for coccidioidomycosis, 205
Food
  contaminated, and communicable disease, 217
  as primary prevention, in school setting, 170
Fractures, 86, 160
Functional Health Status Inventory, 116–119

G

Gastrointestinal system
  aging and, implications for health in, 111–112
  health hazards and, 173
  health problems with
    in children, 85
    in school setting, 160
Gastrointestinal upset, drug classifications and, 10
Genitourinary system, health problems with, in school setting, 160
Geopolitical communities, 152
Girls, urinalysis screening in, 67
Glucose, urine tests for, normal values for, 114
Glucose tolerance test (GTT), normal values for, 114
Goals, in health education process, 11
Gonorrhea, 205
Group development
  stages of, 41
  tasks of, by stage and related nursing process component, 41
Group process, 2, 40–41
Group therapy, for substance abuse, 232–233
Growth, in children, 84
Growth deficiency, in fetus, 225
Growth patterns, 72

H

Hair, aging and, implications for health in, 111
Hallucinogen(s), 225–227, 233
Handicapping conditions, in school setting, 172
Hand-mouth movement, in children, anticipatory guidance for, 64
Hands
  optical placing of hands reflex, 69
  plantar grasp reflex, 69
Hantavirus, 206

Hay fever, 160
Head trauma, and family violence, 242
Headache, 86
Health
  attitudes about, and health education process, 12
  relationship to education, 159
Health Assessment
  in school setting, 162–169
  in work setting, 181–188
Health Assessment and Intervention Guide, for community client, 150–151
Health Assessment and Intervention Planning Guide, for family client, 137–144
Health Assessment Guide
  for adult client, 92–100
  for older clients, 123–130
Health care
  attitudes about, and health education process, 12
  lack of, and family violence, 243
Health education
  nutritional assessment and, 4
  in school setting, 170
Health education encounter
  evaluation of, 17
  outcome objectives for, 12–13
  planning and implementing of, 16
  tasks involved in, 11
Health education process, 2, 11
Health hazards, in occupational settings, 173–175
Health history, 72. *See also* Prior health history
Health Intervention Planning Guide, for community client, 152–158
Health learning needs, and health education process, 11

Health problems
  in children, 85–88
  in school setting, 160
Health promotion, 3, 61, 161
Health screening. *See also* Screening
  in school setting, 171
Health status. *See* Functional Health Status Inventory
Health system dimension, 2
Health-promotive nursing diagnoses, 45
Health-related literature, 45
Hearing loss, health hazards and, 174–175
Hearing problems, in children, 86
Hearing screening, for children, 67
Heart murmurs, 160
Heat, as occupational hazard, 174
Heat stroke, health hazards and, 174
Heavy metals, 53–54
  as occupational hazard, 174
Hematocrit, screening in children, 67
Hematopoietic system, health problems with, in school setting, 160
Hemoglobin
  normal values for, 114
  screening in children, 67
Hemophilia, in school setting, 160
Hemophilus influenzae type B vaccine (HiB), recommendations for administration, 67
Hepatitis, 160
Hepatitis A, 206
  school readmission guidelines for, 161
Hepatitis B, 206–207
Hepatitis B vaccine, recommendations for administration, 68
Hepatitis C, 207
Hepatitis D (Delta), 207

Hepatitis E, 208
Herpes simplex virus (HSV), 208–209
HIV. *See* Human immunodeficiency virus (HIV)
Home, avenues of escape from, 191
Home health clients, functional ability of, 116–119
Home Health Nursing Assessment, 25–30
Home Safety Inventory
 for children, 21–23
 for older adults, 21, 24
Home visit(s), 18
 elements of, 20
Home visit process, 2, 18–24
 advantages of, 18
 personal safety considerations in, 18–19
Homelessness
 and communicable disease, 217
 and family violence, 242
 and substance abuse, 231
Homicide, work-related, 175
Homosexual families, 135
Hospitalization, for cocaine abuse, 232
Housekeeping activities, assessment of, 118
HSV. *See* Herpes simplex virus (HSV)
Human behaviors, and emergence of diseases, 203
Human immunodeficiency virus (HIV), 208
Hurricanes, disaster preparedness for, 191
Hygiene
 in older clients, 131
 poor, and communicable disease, 218
Hyperactivity, 225
Hypercholesterolemics, 10
Hypertension, 160

Hyperthermia, health hazards and, 174
Hypnotherapy, 233
Hypnotics, 10, 225–227, 232
Hypothermia, health hazards and, 174

I

Illness, signs and symptoms of
 atypical symptoms in women, 91
 in children versus adults, 73
Illness prevention, for schoolchildren, 161
Illness prevention services, and children, 61
Immunization history, 72
Immunizations
 for adults, 67–68
 for children, 67–68, 84
 for diphtheria, 67, 132
 influenza, 132
 lack of, and communicable disease, 218
 for older clients, 132
 in school setting, 170
 for tetanus, 67, 132
Immunoglobulin(s)
 for Hepatitis A, 205–206
 for rubella, in pregnant women, 211
 tetanus, 212
Immunologic system, health problems with, in school setting, 160
Immunosuppressive therapy, and communicable disease, 217
Impact stage, 189
Impetigo
 school readmission guidelines for, 161
 in school setting, 160

Impulse control
  and family violence, 242
  and substance abuse, 231
Income, and health education process, 12
Incontinence. *See* Urinary incontinence
Independence activities, in older clients, 132
Infant(s)
  assessment of, 72
  home safety inventory for, 22
  nutritional status of, 73
  reflexes in, 68–70
Infectious agents, preventive measures for, 54
Influenza, 209
  immunization for, 132
  school readmission guidelines for, 161
  in school setting, 160
Influenza vaccine, recommendations for administration, 68
Inhalants, 225–227, 233
Insect bites, and communicable disease, 217
  portals of entry and exit for, 204
Insects, primary preventive measures against, 54–55
Insomnia, and substance abuse, 231
Institutional living, and communicable disease, 217
Instrumental activities of daily living, 118–119
Integumentary system
  aging and, implications for health in, 110–111
  health problems with
    in children, 85–86
    in school setting, 160
Intelligence, assessment of, 121
Interpersonal dimension, 2

Interpersonal skills, in school setting, 171
Intoxication, with psychoactive substance, signs of, 226
Intrauterine growth retardation, in fetus, psychoactive drugs and, 225
IPV. *See* Trivalent inactivated poliovirus vaccine (IPV)
Isoniazid, for tuberculosis, 212
Itraconazole, for coccidioidomycosis, 205

J

Jealousy, of new baby, 87
Joint tenancy, 238
Judgment, assessment of, 121

K

Ketoconazole, for coccidioidomycosis, 205
Kidneys, health hazards and, 174

L

Laboratory tests
  normal values for, in young adult versus older adult clients, 114–115
  and nutritional assessment, 4
Lacerations, 86
Lactate dehydrogenase (LDH), normal values for, 115
Landau reflex, 68
Laryngeal diphtheria, 205
Launching center family, 136
Laundry activities, assessment of, 118

LDH. *See* Lactate dehydrogenase (LDH)
Lead
    as occupational hazard, 174
    primary preventive measures for, 53–54
    screening in children, 67
Lead poisoning, in school setting, 160
Leadership process, 2
Learner, in health education process, 11
Learning ability, assessment of, 121
Learning disabilities, in school setting, 160
    preventing adverse effects of, 172
Learning needs. *See* Health learning needs
Learning objectives
    and breast self-examination, 107
    and testicular self-examination, 109
Learning situation
    elements of, 12
    in health education process, 11, 14–15
Leg cramps, in children, 86
Legg-Calve-Perthes disease, in school setting, 160
Leisure activities, 127, 140, 155, 165, 185, 231
Leukemia, in school setting, 160
Leukocytes, normal values for,
Lice, in school setting, 160
Life resolution issues, in older clients, 132
Lifestyle, 79–80
Limit, setting, and discipline, 71
Literature, as data source in cultural assessment, 45
Living conditions, crowded, and communicable disease, 217

Loss, recent, and substance abuse, 231
Low birth weight, 225
Lower respiratory infections, in school setting, 160
Lung cancer, health hazards and, 173–175
Lung irradiation, health hazards and, 174
Lungs, health hazards and, 174
Lyme disease, 209
    in school setting, 160
Lymphatic cancer, health hazards and, 174
Lymphocytes, normal values for, 114

M

Malnutrition, and communicable diseases, 218
Maturation, assessment of
    in adult client, 93
    in children, 76
Measles, 209–210
    school readmission guidelines for, 161
    in school setting, 160
Measles, mumps, rubella vaccine (MMR)
    for measles, 209
    recommendations for administration, 67
Medication history, and nutritional assessment, 4, 9
Memory, assessment of, 121
Men, testicular self-examination for, 109
Meningitis
    meningococcal, school readmission guidelines for, 161
    in school setting, 160

Men's health, assessment of
  cultural influences and, 91
  general considerations in, 90–91
  review of systems in, 90
Mental health problems, clients with, functional ability of. *See* Functional Health Status Inventory
Mental illness
  and family violence, 242
  and substance abuse, 231
Mental retardation, in school setting, 160
Mercury, as occupational hazard, 174–175
Metal fume fever, health hazards and, 175
Methadone, for opioids abuse, 232
Microcephaly, perinatal exposure to psychoactive drugs and, 225
MMR. *See* Measles, mumps, rubella vaccine (MMR)
Mobility limitation, in older clients, 133
Modes of transmission. *See* Transmission, modes of
Modesty, physical, respecting in assessment of children, 72
Money management activities, assessment of, 119
Mononucleosis, infectious
  school readmission guidelines for, 161
  in school setting, 160
Morbidity rates, 153
Moro reflex, 68–69
Mortality rates, 152
Motivation, in health education process, 12
Mumps, 210
  school readmission guidelines for, 161
  in school setting, 160

Musculoskeletal injury, health hazards and, 175
Musculoskeletal system
  aging and, implications for health and, 112–113
  health problems with
    in children, 86
    in school setting, 160
Mycobacterium tuberculosis, 212. *See also* Tuberculosis
Mycoplasma pneumonia, school readmission guidelines for, 161
Myocardial infarction, atypical symptoms for, in women, 91

N

Nails, aging and, implications for health in, 111
Narcotics Anonymous, 232
Nasal cancer, health hazards and, 175
Natural environment, safety hazards in, 58
Neck, asymmetrical tonic reflex of, 68
Neck righting reflex, 69
Negative emotional climate, and family violence, 242
Negativity, in children, anticipatory guidance for, 65
Neglect
  in children, 73, 234
  in elderly, 236–237
  in older clients, 133
Negotiation, in group development, tasks involved in, 41
Neighborhood/Community Safety Inventory, 57–60
Neisseria gonorrhoeae, 205. *See also* Gonorrhea
Neonatal history, 72

Nervous system, health hazards and, 174
Neurological system
 aging and, implications for health in, 113
 health problems with, in children, 86–87
Neurophysical development
 of adolescents and adults, 89–90
 in children, 62–63
Newborn(s)
 Postpartum/Newborn Visit Intervention Checklist, 105–106
 reflexes in, 68–70
Nickel, as occupational hazard, 175
Nicotine, 225–227, 233
Night terrors, in children
 anticipatory guidance for, 66
 nursing interventions for, 87
Noise
 and chronic diseases, 222
 as occupational hazard, 175
 primary preventive measures for, 54
Noncompliance, and chronic diseases, 223
Nondisaster stage, 189
Nuclear conjugal families, 135
Nursing care, in school setting, 161
Nursing diagnoses
 health-promotive, 45, 51
 positive, 45, 51
 problem-focused, 45, 51
Nursing process, 2
 components of, in group development, 41
Nutrition
 in children, 79
  primary preventive interventions for, 84
 and health promotion, 3
 in older clients, 131
 in school setting, 170
Nutritional Assessment Guide, 4–9
Nutritional history
 of adolescents, 72
 of children, 72
Nutritional status
 of children, 73–74
 drug classifications and, 10

O

Objectives
 in health education encounter, 12–13
 in health education process, 11
Occupation, 12, 140
Occupational activities, 119
Occupational health, assessment of, general considerations in, 180
Occupational risk
 and chronic diseases, 222
 and communicable disease, 217
Occupational settings. *See also* Work setting
 health hazards in, 173–175
Odyssey House, 232
Older clients, 110–134. *See also* Adult clients
 aging and, implications for health in, 110–113
 assessment of, general considerations in, 115
 Health Assessment Guide for, 123–130
 home safety inventory for, 21, 24
 normal laboratories values for, changes in, 114–115
 primary prevention for, 131–132
 rest and exercise and, 132
 secondary prevention for, 132–134

Operation, in group development, tasks involved in, 41
Opioid antagonists, for opioids abuse, 232
Opioids, 225–227, 232
Opportunistic infections, related to AIDS, in school setting, 160
Optical placing of hands reflex, 69
OPV. *See* Trivalent oral poliovirus vaccine (OPV)
Oral contraceptives, 10
Orientation
  assessment of, 122
  in group development, tasks involved in, 41
Otitis externa, in school setting, 160
Otitis media, in school setting, 160
Outcome objectives, for health education encounter, 12–13
Overweight, and chronic diseases, 222

P

Pain, in older clients, 133
Palmar grasp reflex, 69
Parachute reflex, 69
Parents, education of, 84
PCP, intoxication, signs of, 226
Pediculosis, school readmission guidelines for, 161
Peer pressure
  and chronic diseases, 222
  and communicable disease, 217
  and substance abuse, 231
Penicillin, 205, 211–212
Peptic ulcer, in school setting, 160
Perception, assessment of, 122
Perinatal period, exposure to psychoactive substances in, effects of, 225
Personal safety considerations, in home visit process, 18–19

Pertussis, 210
  school readmission guidelines for, 161
  in school setting, 160
Pesticides, as occupational hazard, 175
Pharmacological therapy, for substance abuse, 232
Pharyngotonsillar diphtheria, 205
Phenylketonuria, screening for, in children, 67
Phoenix House, 232
Physical abuse
  in children, 234–235
  in elderly, 237
Physical dimension, 2
Physical environment
  in Child Health Assessment Guide, 78
  in health education process, 12
Physical examination
  of adult client, 94–95
  of children, 72, 77–78
    pace of, 72
    restraining in, 72
  and nutritional assessment, 4
Physical findings, variations in, in assessment of children, 72
Physical indications
  of child abuse, 234–235
  of elder abuse, 236–237
  of spouse abuse, 236
Physical limitations, and chronic diseases, 222
Physical modesty, respecting in assessment of children, 72
Physiologic function, 76, 93, 124
Placement decisions, in workplace, 176
Plantar grasp reflex, 69
Plants
  poisonous, 52
  preventive measures for, 55
Platelets, normal values for, 114

Pneumococcal pneumonia, school readmission guidelines for, 161
Pneumonia
  school readmission guidelines for, 161
  in school setting, 160
Pneumonia vaccine
  for older clients, 132
  recommendations for administration, 68
Poisonous plants, common, 52
Poisons, primary preventive measures against, 55
Poliomyelitis, 210–211
Poliovirus vaccine, recommendations for administration, 67
Political activities, community health nurses and, 224
Political process, 2
Pollutants, environmental, and chronic diseases, 222
Pollution. See Air pollution; Water pollution
Population(s)
  in community assessment, composition of, 152
  in disaster setting, vulnerable, 199
Population groups, 148, 150, 219–221, 228, 239, 244
  identification of problems in, 123
Portals of entry, for communicable diseases, 204
Portals of exit, for communicable diseases, 204
Positive nursing diagnoses, 45
Postpartum/Newborn Visit Intervention Checklist, 105–106
Potassium, normal values for, 114
Power allocation, and family violence, 242
PPD. See Tuberculin skin test (PPD)

Predisaster stage, 189
Pregnancy
  and communicable disease, 217
  and family violence, 242
  Postpartum/Newborn Visit Intervention Checklist, 105–106
  Prenatal Care Checklist during, 101–104
  in school setting, 160
  and sexual abuse of children, 236
  for substance abuse, 231
Pregnancy history, 72
Prematurity, 225
Prenatal Care Checklist, 101–104
Preschool children
  family with, developmental tasks of, 135
  home safety inventory for, 22–23
  nutritional status of, 74
Prescription drugs, and substance abuse, 231
Primary prevention, 2
  for air pollution, 55–56
  for animals, 54–55
  for children, 84
  for environmental hazards, 53–56
  for heavy metals, 53–54
  for infectious agents, 54
  for insects, 54–55
  for lead, 53–54
  for noise, 54
  for older clients, 131–132
  for plants, 55
  for poisons, 55
  for radiation, 53
  in school setting, 170–171
  for substance abuse, 224
  for water pollution, 56
Prior health history, 72
Problem solving ability, assessment of, 122

Problem-focused diagnoses, 45, 75
Process dimension, 3–41
　components of, 2
Prostatic cancer, health hazards and, 174
Prostitution, and substance abuse, 232
Protein, urine tests for, normal values for, 114
Psychoactive substances, 225–227, 231–233
Psychological dimension, 2
Psychological environment, 79
　safety hazards in, assessment of, 59
Psychological indications
　of child abuse, 234–235
　of elder abuse, 236–237
　of spouse abuse, 236
Psychological literature, 45
Psychomotor ability, 122
Psychosocial development
　of adolescents and adults, 89–90
　in children, 62–63
Psychosocial interventions, for inhalants abuse, 233
Psychotherapy, for substance abuse, 232–233
Pulmonary hantavirus, 206

Q

Qualitative data, 148–149
Quantitative data, 148

R

Radiation
　as occupational hazard, 175
　preventive measures for, 53

Radiation sickness, health hazards and, 175
Reaction time, assessment of, 122
Readmission guidelines, for conditions warranting exclusion from school, 160–161
Reality orientation, 134
Reconstruction stage, 189–190
Recreation activities
　assessment of, 119
　high-risk, and chronic diseases, 223
Referral(s)
　for alcohol abuse, 232
　and Resource File Entry Form, 37
　in school setting, 171
Referral process, 2, 32
Reflective dimension, 2
Reflex(es). *See also* specific reflexes
　infant and newborn, 68–70
Relaxation training, 233
Religion, and health education process, 12
Renal system, health hazards and, 174
Representative payee, 238
Reproductive system
　aging and, implications for health in, 112
　health hazards and, 174
　health problems with, in school setting, 160
Researcher, community health nurse role as, 218
Residential programs, for substance abuse, 232–233
Resource File Entry Form, 37–39
Respiratory disease, viral, school readmission guidelines for, 161
Respiratory infection(s)
　in children, 85
　in school setting, 160

INDEX **267**

Respiratory system
  aging and, implications for health in, 111
  health hazards and, 173–175
  health problems with
    in children, 85
    in school setting, 160
Respite care, 84
Rest, 80, 97
  in older clients, primary prevention strategies for, 132
Retirement, families in, developmental tasks of, 136
Rights, denial of, in elderly, 237
Rimantadine, for influenza, 209
Risk factor inventory(ies)
  for chronic diseases, 219–221
  for family violence, 239–241
  for substance abuse, 228–230
  for suicide, 244–246
Risk factor modification strategies
  for chronic disease, 222–223
  for communicable disease, 217–218
  for family violence, 242–243
  for substance abuse, 231–232
  for suicide, 247
Role model, community health nurse role as, 218
Rolling over, in children, anticipatory guidance for, 64
Rooting reflex, 69
Rubella, 211
  school readmission guidelines for, 161
  in school setting, 160
Rules, children's understanding of, and discipline, 71

S

Safety
  in children, 84
  in home visit process, 18–19
  in older clients, 131
  in school setting, 170
  in work setting, 180
Safety hazards
  and chronic diseases, 222
  in neighborhoods/communities, 58–60
  in work setting, 180
Safety inventory, neighborhood/community, 57–60
Safety problems, 60
Sanitary conditions, poor, and communicable disease, 217
Scabies
  school readmission guidelines for, 161
  in school setting, 160
Scarlet fever
  school readmission guidelines for, 161
  in school setting, 160
School anxiety, anticipatory guidance for, 66
School community nurse, community health nurse as, 161
School exclusion
  conditions typically warranting, readmission guidelines for, 160–161
  as primary prevention, in school setting, 170
School nurse, community health nurse as, 161
School nurse practitioner, community health nurse as, 161
School setting, 159–172
  community health nurse in, roles of, 161
  health assessment in, 162–169
  health problems encountered in, acute and chronic, 160

School setting (cont.)
  nursing care in, focus groups of, 161
  prevention measures in, 170–172
School-age children
  families with, developmental tasks of, 135–136
  home safety inventory for, 23
  nutritional status of, 74
Schoolchildren, health of, 161
Scoliosis
  in school setting, 160
  screening in children, 67
Screening
  for children, 67
  lack of, and chronic diseases, 223
  in school setting, 171
  in work setting, 180
Secondary prevention, 2
  for older clients, 132–134
  in school setting, 171
Sedatives, 10, 225–227, 232
Sedentary lifestyle, and chronic diseases, 223
Seizure disorders, in school setting, 160
Self-care practices
  and chronic diseases, 223
  of women, with caregiver responsibilities, 91
Self-esteem, poor, in children, 88
Self-help groups, for substance abuse, 232–233
Self-image
  and communicable disease, 217
  and family violence, 242
  in school setting, 170
  and substance abuse, 231
Sensory loss, in older clients, 133
Separation anxiety, anticipatory guidance for, 66
Setting, of learning situation, 12

Sexual abuse
  in children, 235–236
  in elderly, 237
Sexual activity, unsafe
  and chronic diseases, 222
  and communicable disease, 218
Sexual contact transmission, of communicable diseases, portals of entry and exit for, 204
Sexual development, anticipatory guidance for, 66
Sexual dominance, and family violence, 243
Sexuality issues, in older clients, 127
Sexually transmitted diseases
  in school setting, 160
  and sexual abuse of children, 236
Shelter living, and communicable disease, 217
Shopping activities, assessment of, 118
Sibling rivalry
  anticipatory guidance for, 66
  in children, 87–88
Sickle cell disease
  in school setting, 160
  screening in children, 67
Single-parent families, 135
Sitting, in children, anticipatory guidance for, 64
Skin
  aging and, implications for health in, 110
  breakdown of, in older clients, 132
  health hazards and, 175
Skin cancer, health hazards and, 175
Skin ulcers, health hazards and, 174
Smoke detectors, 191
Smoking, and chronic diseases, 223
Social activities, assessment of, 119

Social dimension, 2
Social environment, 79
　safety hazards in, 59
Social interactions, assessment of, 122
Social isolation
　and family violence, 242
　in older clients, 133
　and substance abuse, 231
Social literature, 45
Social mores
　and chronic diseases, 222
　and communicable disease, 217
　and family violence, 242
Social services, 232
Societal changes, and emergence of diseases, 203
Sociodrama, 233
Sodium, normal values for, 114
Specific gravity test, normal values for, 114
Speech, in children
　anticipatory guidance for, 65
　delayed, 87
Speech defect, in children, 87
Spitting up, in children, 85
Spontaneous abortion, 225
Spouse abuse
　indications of, 236
　risk factors for, 239
Sprains, 86, 160
Standing, in children, anticipatory guidance for, 64
Startle reflex, 68–69
Stepfamilies, 135
Steroids, 10
Stillbirth, 225
Strep throat
　school readmission guidelines for, 161
　in school setting, 160
Streptococcus infections, school readmission guidelines for, 161

Stress
　and chronic diseases, 222
　and communicable disease, 217
　and family violence, 242
　as occupational hazard, 175
　and substance abuse, 231
　in women, from caretaking responsibilities, 91
Substance abuse, 224–233
　and chronic diseases, 222
　and communicable disease, 218
　and family violence, 243
　risk factor modification strategies for, 231–232
　treatment modalities for, 232–233
Substance Abuse Risk Factor Inventory, 228–230
Substitution, 233
Sucking reflex, 69
Suicide, risk factor modification strategies for, 247
Suicide Risk Factor Inventory, 244–246
Sun exposure
　and chronic diseases, 223
　as occupational hazard, 175
Sunburn, health hazards and, 174
Supervisor, community health nurse as, 161
Supporting reaction reflex, 70
Supportive therapy, 233
Symptoms, of illness
　atypical symptoms in women, 91
　in children versus adults, 73
Synanon, 232
Syphilis, 211–212
Systems. *See* Body systems

T

Tantrums, in children, 88
Teaching strategies
　for breast self-examination, 107

Teaching strategies (*cont.*)
  in health education process, 11–12
  for testicular self-examination, 109
Teenagers, families with, developmental tasks of, 136
Teething, in children, anticipatory guidance for, 64
Temperature extremes, and chronic diseases, 222
Tertiary prevention, 2
  in school setting, 172
Testicular self-examination (TSE), 109
Tetanus, 212
  immunizations for, 67
  in older client, 132
Tetanus, diphtheria vaccine (Td), 212
  recommendations for administration, 67
Tetanus antitoxin, 212
Tetanus immunoglobulin (TIg), 212
Tetracycline, for chlamydia, 204
Therapeutic communities, for opioids abuse, 232
Thyroid, aging and, implications for health in, 113
Thyroid disorders, in school setting, 160
Thyroid-stimulating hormone (TSH), normal values for, 114
Thyroxine (T_4), normal values for, 114
Tinea corporis
  school readmission guidelines for, 161
  in school setting, 160
Toddler(s)
  home safety inventory for, 22
  nutritional status of, 74
Toilet training, in children, anticipatory guidance for, 65
Toileting activities, assessment of, 117
Tornado(s), disaster preparedness for, 191
Traction response reflex, 70
Tranquilizers, for alcohol abuse, 232
Transfer activities, assessment of, 117–118
Transmission, modes of, for communicable diseases, 204
Transportation, and personal safety considerations, in home visiting, 18–19
Transposition of great vessels, 225
Trauma
  as occupational hazard, 175
  cumulative, 173
  work-related, 175
Traumatic injury, health hazards and, 175
Travel, and communicable disease, 217
Treatment, in school setting, 171
Treponema pallidum, 211. *See also* Syphilis
Tricyclic antidepressants, for cocaine abuse, 232
Triglycerides, normal values for, 114
Triiodothyronine (T_3), normal values for, 114
Trivalent inactivated poliovirus vaccine (IPV), recommendations for administration, 67
Trivalent oral poliovirus vaccine (OPV), recommendations for administration, 67

TSE. *See* Testicular self-examination (TSE)
TSH. *See* Thyroid-stimulating hormone (TSH)
Tuberculin skin test (PPD), in children, 67
Tuberculosis, 212
Tungsten, as occupational hazard, 175

U

Unacceptable behavior, prevention rather than punishment of, in discipline, 71
Unemployment
 and family violence, 242
 and substance abuse, 231
United States, death in, leading causes of, 218
Universal precautions, for bloodborne diseases, 19–20
Unrealistic expectations
 and family violence, 242
 and substance abuse, 231
Upper respiratory infection
 school readmission guidelines for, 161
 in school setting, 160
Urinalysis, screening in children, 67
Urinary incontinence, in older clients, 132–133
Urinary system, aging and, implications for health in, 112
Urinary tract infection
 in children, 86
 in school setting, 160
Urine tests, normal values for, 114

V

Values testing, in children, anticipatory guidance for, 66
Varicella vaccine, recommendations for administration, 68
Vibration, as occupational hazard, 173
Violence, 234–237
 as occupational hazard, 175
Vision, of children
 problems with, 86
 screening for, 67
Vocational rehabilitation, 232–233
Vomiting, in children, 85
Vulnerable populations, in disaster settings, 199

W

Walking, in children, anticipatory guidance for, 64
Water, contaminated, and communicable disease, 217
Water pollution, 56
Weaning, anticipatory guidance for, 64
Weather, exposure to, as occupational hazard, 174
Weight gain, steroids and, 10
Wellness diagnoses, 75
Withdrawal, 227
Women. *See also* Pregnancy
 breast self-examination for, 107–108
 with caretaking responsibilities
  self-care practices of, 91
  stress of, 91
  and family violence, 91

Women's health
  assessment of
    atypical symptoms and, 91
    general considerations in, 91
  cultural influences on, 91
Work, employees return to, 176
Work Fitness Inventory, 176–179

Work setting, 173–188. *See also* Occupational settings

Z

Zinc oxide, as occupational hazard, 175